Sugar Detox *for Beginners*

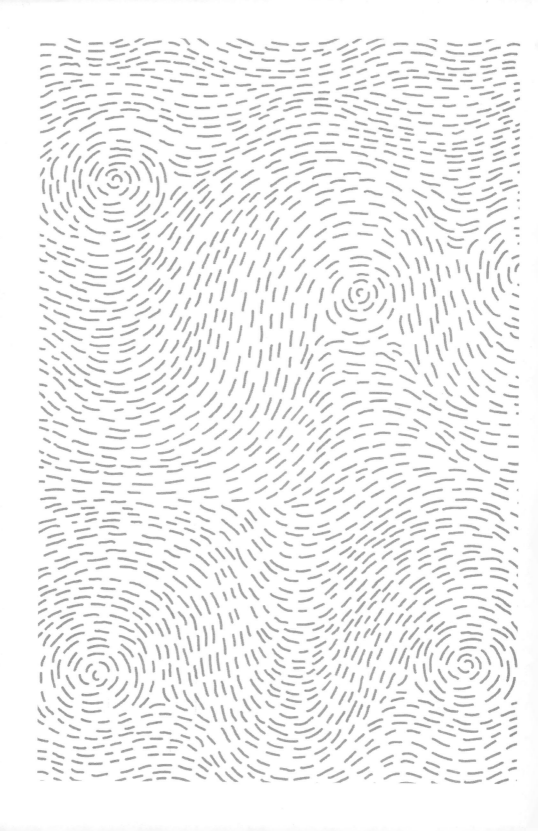

Sugar Detox
for Beginners

YOUR GUIDE TO STARTING
A 21-DAY SUGAR DETOX

DRAKES PRESS

Contents

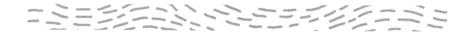

PART ONE

Fundamentals of the Sugar Detox Diet

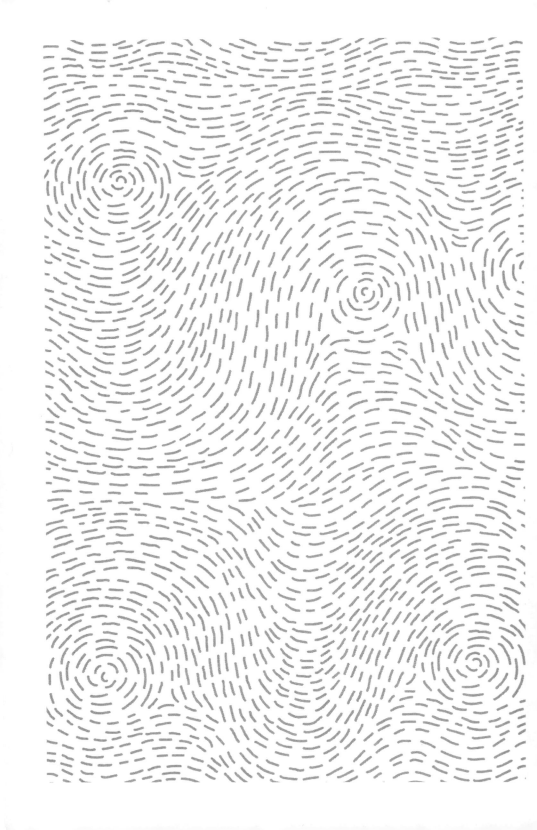

Introduction

Sugar. It might have come on as sweet and harmless, but, like a bad boyfriend or girlfriend, over time it revealed its true colors. You don't like what you see. Or feel.

If the romance is over—if you've had enough of feeling lousy, craving increasing amounts of the sweet stuff, and feeling out of control—you've come to the right place. This book will give you the tools you need to feel well and in control. When you're ready to "detoxify" from sugar, you'll find recipes, inspiration, and information in these pages.

You'll learn to think about your diet in new ways, and to substitute healthful foods and behaviors for those that weren't working for you. This book is designed to offer maximum flexibility and ease—two things you could probably use a lot more of in your life and your diet.

You'll also find information about dealing with special situations or diets that are sugar-free-plus-something-else (kosher, halal, vegetarian). Nothing should stand between you and the life and health you want.

Sugar detoxing should not leave you hungry, fatigued, or moody. Just the opposite: After a few days of careful eating, you should begin to feel revitalized. The longer you refrain from eating sugar, the easier it will likely become. The better you'll feel, and even look. (Sugar's no good for your skin, either, except topically.) Sweet! Or maybe not.

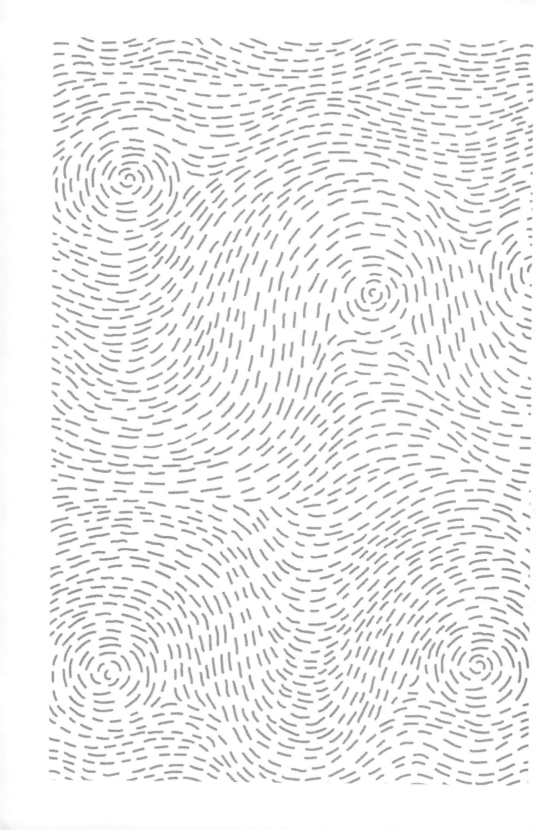

CHAPTER 1

Addicted to Sugar

Honey. Ah, sugar, sugar. In some ways, not much has changed since the Archies reached the top of the music charts with this sweet, bouncy number circa 1969. Husbands and wives still call each other "honey." Kids are "sweetie," and Mom, perhaps, still asks her special someone for "some sugar." Oh, but those are just expressions, aren't they?

There's no doubt that we're hooked on the sweet stuff. Sugar—and its close relatives, honey (which, contrary to popular perception, offers little to no nutritional value), corn syrup, molasses, and even fructose—is big business. And, since the 1940s, the sugar industry has been doing all it can to ensure the favorability of its product in the eyes of the public. Lately, people have been wising up. But old habits can be hard to break. Addictions, of course, are even harder.

You may have grown up thinking that sugar was perfectly harmless, or even wholesome. Many Americans and Europeans still begin their days with the sugar-sweetened cereals or chocolate milk they enjoyed in childhood. Perhaps you have graduated to sweetened coffee drinks, muffins or Danishes, or—heaven help us!—cola. (Oh, and contrary to another popular belief, orange juice, beneficial though it is, contains lots of sugar. You're better off with a whole orange or grapefruit. Bran muffins, fruit shakes, and instant oatmeal aren't nutritional bargains, either.)

As the day progresses, you might reach for the "quick energy" (actually a myth) of candy bars, the office donut cart, or "energy bars" (most of which are little better, if at all, than candy). Chances are, dinner ends with a sweet dessert—to say nothing of the various snacks you might have consumed throughout the day.

No wonder the World Health Organization calls diabetes "an emerging global epidemic." Diabetes and its complications are a major cause of death worldwide—and, as you may have heard, the prevalence of type 2 diabetes (the kind that is usually acquired rather than inherited) among children and adults has been growing by leaps and bounds.

Worse, sugar is addictive: The more you consume, the more you'll crave. That, of course, will drive you to eat ever-greater quantities of the sweet stuff. And then what? Well, then you're at higher-than-average risk not only for diabetes, but also for many other diseases. Sugar, according to celebrity dermatologist Nicholas Perricone, MD, causes inflammation—which, in turn, can give rise to many maladies. But that's not all. That same inflammatory property that can make us sick also ages our skin prematurely. That's right: sugar can actually cause wrinkles!

The flip side? Just as sugar can weaken our bodies and age us, avoiding sugar can help us enjoy better health and greater beauty. Difficult? It can be. But this book helps make "sugar detoxing" less painful than you might think. Let's start by playing a little game. How much of a problem is sugar for you? To find out, try your hand at the following quiz. Go on—it's fun!

QUIZ: ARE YOU ADDICTED TO SUGAR?

1. I consume _____ soft drinks ("cola," "soda," "pop") during a typical day.
   A. No
   B. One
   C. Two or three
   D. Four or more

2. I believe a glass of orange juice is:
   A. Essential every morning
   B. A bad idea, because OJ, even though it has lots of vitamin C, is loaded with sugar
   C. Not as healthful as a whole orange or grapefruit (either whole or juiced)
   D. A great afternoon pick-me-up

3. I don't eat as many vegetables as I should because:
   A. They're too hard to prepare. Donuts, candy, and fast food are ready when I am!
   B. I want to enjoy life—and healthful food isn't as much fun as the other kind!
   C. What are you talking about? I eat plenty of vegetables.
   D. I'm not sure why not. I mean to.

4. I read product labels:
   A. Always
   B. Sometimes
   C. Nah
   D. The print is too small. Who do they make these things for?

5. When I do read a product label, I look for:
   A. Sugar
   B. Cane sugar
   C. Barley malt
   D. All kinds of sugar—cane, brown sugar, honey, molasses, fructose, barley malt, and so on

6. "Hidden sugars" can be found in:
   A. Soups
   B. Packaged salad dressings
   C. Bread
   D. Just about anything

7. When I crave something sweet, I want:
   A. Fruit
   B. Chocolate
   C. Pudding or yogurt
   D. Ice cream

8. When I think about detoxing, I feel:
   A. Excited
   B. A little apprehensive or doubtful
   C. Terrified
   D. Confident. It may be tough, but I know I can do it!

9. When I feel frustrated, bored, or sad, I find myself turning to sweet treats for comfort:
   A. Sometimes
   B. Often
   C. Pretty much all the time
   D. Never. I look for constructive ways to deal with problems or bad feelings.

10. Most of the time, I eat sweet treats when I am:
    A. Alone
    B. At social functions, including business events
    C. At work
    D. Traveling
    E. At dinner with friends, or on rare special occasions, such as my birthday

Scoring

Best answers: 1. A; 2. B or C; 3. C, although any answer can represent one reason you might be reading this book; 4. A (but the print often *is* too small to read comfortably!); 5. D; 6. D; 7. and 8. only you can answer these questions, of course. We hope to provide recipes or at least substitution ideas and strategies to help stem those cravings. Fear, apprehension, self-confidence, and excitement are all valid ways to feel about the prospect of minimizing your body's dependence on sugar; 9. D; 10. E.

But you don't even have to "know the score" to know whether sugar is a bigger part of your life than it needs to be. Think carefully about your answers to these questions. Are you addicted to sugar—and, if so, how badly? The answer should be plain.

THE SCIENCE BEHIND SUGAR ADDICTION

Like caffeine, sugar is believed to be addictive. If you've ever tried to kick the caffeine habit or spent time around someone who hasn't had his morning mug of coffee, you'll understand the comparison. Sugar is, in some ways, more insidious than caffeine, or even nicotine, in that you don't have to drink coffee to live (despite what you might think!). You do, of course, have to eat, and sugar can be—and indeed is—found anywhere and everywhere. It's part of most societal celebrations, too. Think birthday cake, the champagne toast (alcohol is loaded with sugar), celebration dinners, and even Sunday brunch.

Sugar is far from the harmless little enjoyment it was once believed to be. According to a recent report on WebMD.com, the human species is hardwired to crave, or at least enjoy, sweet tastes. It's not hard to understand why: In ancient days, sweet meant something was safe to eat (as was the case for, say, most fruits), and full of enough calories to sustain a Neanderthal until his or her next meal—whenever that might arrive. Sweet tastes, according to

WebMD, even have the power to alleviate pain, at least in infants. Although science so far has shown reluctance to draw conclusions about whether sugar addiction is psychologically or physically based, apparently some animal studies do concede that a theory of physical addiction might well be borne out.

Experiments using laboratory rats and mice have yielded interesting findings. You may remember reading that a recent study concluded that Oreo cookies were as addictive as cocaine.[1] That's because lab rats running a maze went for the cookies much more often than rice cake rewards. (Surprising? Probably not!) Other studies using mice came up with equally interesting findings.[2]

According to many anecdotal, and a few scientific, observations, sugar would seem to be psychologically addictive as well. Luckily, however, "withdrawal" symptoms seem to be relegated to the emotional realm. That is, a sugar addict may become cranky or even weepy as a result of her diet, but she will not likely die or convulse as a result of sugar deprivation. This is obviously good news for you! WebMD points out another unhappy consequence of addiction, whether physical or psychological: the addict will continue to engage in the unhealthful behavior even when he sees that it is having a bad effect on his health or the way others see him.

We believe that sugar will one day be considered a mild poison. Perhaps it will even be illegal someday! But for now, sugar is here to stay.

The good news? We can make new choices, starting today. Unhealthful eating habits don't have to stick around. Not at all.

Not sure where to start? Don't worry—this book will serve as your guide. Here are ten tips to get you going.

TEN TIPS FOR BEATING SUGAR CRAVINGS

1. Hunger and inadequate nutrition are the principal causes of cravings. Keep yourself well nourished, consuming small "mini meals" that contain protein throughout the day.
2. A big part of one's dependence on fast, prepared, or snack foods has to do with the readiness of such foods. Anticipate your need to eat, and cook before you're hungry. Keep hard-boiled eggs, plain yogurt, celery, bok choi, bell pepper strips, or green apples on hand to combat cravings.

---

1. Forbes.com, "Why Oreo Cookies Are as Addictive as Cocaine to Your Brain," by Alice G. Walton.
2. See *The Sugar Addict's Total Recovery Program*, by Kathleen DesMaisons, PhD, for a discussion of C57 mice.

3. Remember that the craving will reach a peak and then spiral back down. If you can keep away from sugar for three whole days, you'll almost certainly find that you crave it less. The longer you keep away from it, the less you'll find you miss it. You might even kick the craving once and for all!

4. If you must eat something sweet, remember that the joy is usually in the first few bites. Taste it, then toss it (or give it away).

5. If it helps just to know "it's there," store a tempting treat in the freezer. But know yourself. If you're reasonably sure you won't be able to resist the temptation, throw it out or give it away—quickly!

6. Substitute. Prepare sugar-free versions of old favorites. (See the Desserts chapter for recipes.) Apple pie, for instance, can be prepared without sugar. So can whipped cream (although, alas, it still contains plenty of fat).

7. Take a hike—or at least a walk. When the craving hits, tell yourself you're going to do something healthful instead, then get out into the sunshine. This is a win-win, of course, because you're getting beneficial exercise at the same time that you're fighting against indulgence.

8. Delay gratification. If you're cutting down rather than cutting out, remind yourself of an upcoming occasion on which you plan to indulge.

9. Don't get started. When you shop for groceries, do not buy tempting foods. Not only do you not need them, but no one else who lives with you does, either. If they're not in your home in the first place, they can't call to you.

10. Use a tiny touch of stevia. Although we find most artificial sweeteners troubling, so far stevia looks OK. Be advised, however, that while it has enjoyed years of popularity in other countries, it has only recently been cleared for use in the United States.

Ready to jump in? Let's get started.

CHAPTER 2

Starting Your Sugar Detox

Needless to say, when you are embarking on a sugar-detox diet, you'll need to avoid … wait for it … sugar! But as you've seen, that's not always as easy as it sounds. Many packaged foods—too many to list here—contain hidden sugars, and even relatively healthful fruits and vegetables—such as sweet potatoes, corn, oranges, and bananas—are packed with it.

Adding to potential confusion, "sugar-free" can mean different things to different people. Some cookbooks are billed as completely sugar-free—but they use honey, maple syrup, or date sugar in place of table sugar! For other diet-book writers, bread, pasta, and dairy products fall under the "sugar-free" heading.

This book strives to reduce your sugar intake without depriving you of the nutrients contained in many fruits, vegetables, and other foods. The recipes in this book don't use grain, for instance—but remember moderation. Eat what you love—on occasion and in moderate quantities.

Tip: Cookbooks for diabetics are full of sugar-free recipes, of course. Just take care when it comes to using artificial sweeteners.

The following lists will help you navigate the sometimes-muddy waters of sugar detoxing. Pay special attention to the list of foods to enjoy. When you're feeling deprived, it will become like a secret weapon. Of course, you should look at the *other* list carefully, too—foods to avoid. It will help you steer clear of traps that you didn't even know were there.

FOODS TO AVOID

This list can feel a little heartbreaking. So instead of thinking about what you'll miss, think about how much better you'll feel (and look; as you've already read, sugar is responsible for the inflammation that causes wrinkles). Make sure to turn quickly to "Foods to Enjoy." That might take away some of the sting!

The Obvious:

- Ice cream and gelato
- Most granitas
- Most sherbets
- Frozen yogurt
- Presweetened yogurt, including the kind with fruit, honey, or cereal that you stir in
- Pudding, including rice pudding, custard, and flan
- Cake
- Cookies
- Brownies
- Candy

Fruits and Vegetables:

- Bananas*
- Sweet potatoes*
- Butternut squash*
- White potatoes (For a different take on white potatoes, see Kathleen DesMaisons's *The Sugar Addict's Total Recovery Program*.)
- Corn
- Beets
- Parsnips*
- Carrots*
- Peas*
- Beets
- Pineapple*
- Watermelon
- Dried fruit (Be wary not only of banana chips and dried pineapple, obviously, but also of prunes, cranberries, raisins, and dates.)
- Dried vegetables

* These foods, while high in sugar content, also contain vital nutrients. You should be able to enjoy them on occasion.

Bread and Grains:

- Bread
- Donuts
- Bagels
- Muffins
- Crullers
- Croissants
- English muffins
- Rice, including brown rice (Again, Dr. DesMaisons takes a different view.)
- Pasta, including whole grain
- Stuffing

Sweeteners:

- Sugar (of course), white and brown; cane sugar
- Evaporated cane juice
- Demerara sugar
- Honey
- Molasses
- Corn syrup
- Maple syrup
- Fructose
- Barley malt
- Rice syrup
- Agave nectar
- Aspartame

Cereals:

- Frosted cereals
- Many prepared cold cereals (For specifics, you'll want to check labels.)
- Muesli
- Granola
- Presweetened instant oatmeal

Beverages:

- Soft drinks
- Most soy milk
- Most almond milk
- Condensed milk
- Most fruit juice (Grapefruit is OK.)
- Most fruit-vegetable blends
- Alcohol: wine, beer, liquor (All of it contains unhealthful amounts of sugar.)

Condiments:

- Ketchup
- Honey-sweetened mustard (In fact, exercise caution with all mustards; check the label for telltale signs of sugar: fructose, corn syrup, honey, etc.)
- Jellies and jams
- Syrups

FOODS TO ENJOY

Just about any green vegetable and many fruits, such as:

- Spinach
- Snow peas
- Kale
- Zucchini
- Summer squash
- Spaghetti squash
- Broccoli
- Asparagus
- Brussels sprouts
- Green apples
- Pears
- Snow peas
- Pea tendrils
- Arugula
- Collard greens

- Broccolini (also known as "baby broccoli") or broccoli rabe
- Mushrooms
- Lettuce
- Tomatoes, all varieties
- Cucumbers
- Cauliflower
- Grapefruit
- Strawberries
- Blueberries
- Raspberries
- Peppers (all kinds and colors)
- Radishes
- Lettuce
- Bok choi
- Red, green, or Savoy cabbage
- Radicchio
- Leeks
- Onions
- Scallions (also known as "green onions")
- Shallots
- Avocados (and most guacamoles)
- Watercress
- Honeydew melon
- Cantaloupe

Herbs, spices, and flavoring agents:

- Fresh lemon or unsweetened lemon juice
- Fresh lime or unsweetened lime juice
- Vinegar
- Garlic
- Parsley
- Basil
- Pepper, black or white
- Cayenne pepper
- Red pepper flakes
- Paprika
- Cinnamon

- Cilantro (also known as coriander)
- Ginger
- Dill weed
- Mint
- Rosemary
- Oregano
- Sage
- Saffron
- Thyme
- Soy sauce[†] (Take care, however, not to overuse, as soy sauce can be high in sodium and usually contains small amounts of sugar and wheat; it can also contain genetically modified organisms [GMOs].)

Note: Herbs and spices can be fresh or dried.

Protein:

- Lean chicken
- Turkey
- Fish
- Beef
- Pork
- Sugar-free turkey bacon
- Eggs
- Feta cheese (in moderation)[‡]
- Cottage or farmer cheese[‡]
- Ricotta[‡]
- Plain, unsweetened yogurt[‡]
- Beans, including lentils, pinto beans, lima beans, black beans, adzukis, and navy beans
- Bean products such as hummus or falafel
- Nuts, including almonds, peanuts, pecans, cashews, macadamias, pistachios, and Brazil nuts (unless, of course, you are allergic)
- Sunflower seeds and sugar-free sunflower seed butter
- Pumpkin seeds
- Sugar-free soy nut butter[†]
- Sugar-free peanut butter

- Sugar-free almond or cashew butter (but keep the fat content in mind)
- Tofu
- Edamame[†]
- Soy nuts

Grains and Grain Substitutes:

- Slow-cooked oatmeal, unsweetened
- Quinoa
- Whole barley
- Buckwheat, including buckwheat noodles ("soba") and kasha (Confusingly enough, buckwheat is not a wheat at all!)

Snacks:

- Sugar-free pickles
- Sugar-free coleslaw
- Sugar-free sauerkraut
- Sugar-free applesauce[‡]

Beverages:

- Water (Spring water is recommended.)
- Unsweetened tea (Green tea, in particular, is associated with health benefits, including antioxidants, which help retard the aging process.)
- Unsweetened coffee (This option is not as healthful as the others; also, avoid it if you associate it with donuts, cake, or other sugary treats, or if you have a hard time falling asleep or staying asleep.)
- Plain tomato or green vegetable juice (Avoid beet, red and yellow apple, and other sweet veggie juices, or fruit-and-vegetable blends.)
- Unsweetened milk[‡] (See special note on milk, below.)

[†] If it's important to you not to consume GMOs, check the source of the soybeans by searching online or contacting the company that produces the food in question. It's said that up to 90 percent of soybeans consumed in this country may have been genetically modified.

[‡] Do not consume if doing the three-day detox.

Miscellaneous:

- Olives
- Vegetable oil
- Sesame seeds

Fresh fruits and vegetables need to be cleaned before eating or cooking. The best—and most economical—way is to fill a spray bottle with plain white vinegar, spritz thoroughly, and rinse completely under running water. Voilà!

SPECIAL NOTES

Consider these important tips about the following three common ingredients.

Milk: Milk, long considered the most wholesome of foods (or drinks, at any rate), often contains a startling amount of natural sugar. Cheese is a little better—though hard cheeses, in particular, contain high levels of fat and salt.

Spices: Most spices keep best in the refrigerator. In terms of flavor and color, spices are at their best for the first six months after their jars are opened. That said, most spices can be used safely for a long time. Do remember, though: "When in doubt, throw it out."

Nuts: Although free of sugar, nuts are full of fat. Limit your consumption to a few at a time. Prepare a dish or bag of no more than 10 nuts a day, rather than eating right from the package and losing track of how many you've consumed. You can gain weight from these nutritious, wholesome, and satisfying snacks.

SHOPPING TIPS: WHAT TO STOCK IN YOUR PANTRY OR REFRIGERATOR

When sugar and carb cravings come calling, it's helpful to have an arsenal of healthful ingredients at your disposal. Spices, especially, can be your new best friends. They add interest and variety to meals. Healthful snacks, too, are a must-have.

Spices and condiments:

- Sesame seeds
- Coarse pepper

- White pepper
- Dried parsley
- Dill weed
- Dried onion
- Garlic
- Ginger
- Cinnamon
- Turmeric
- Sugar-free all-purpose seasoning, such as Spike brand (Try to find salt-free Spike, if you can.)
- Soy sauce (But use it in moderation, as it usually contains sugar, as well as wheat.)
- Cooking oil
- White vinegar
- Lemon juice
- Lime juice

Snacks:

- Nuts (Almonds, cashews, pecans, macadamias, Brazil nuts, peanuts, unless allergies are a concern; remember the 10-per-day limit due to high fat content.)
- Olives (Check labels for hidden sugars, and consume in moderation, as these are high in sodium.)
- Feta cheese (only if doing the gradual detox)
- Green (Granny Smith) apples
- Celery
- Cucumbers
- Red bell peppers
- Bok choi cabbage (for quick crunchy snacks)
- Hummus

A few staples:

- High-quality slow-cooking (NOT instant) porridge or oatmeal
- Quinoa*
- Beans of all kinds (Lentils cook fastest.)*

- Eggs (A veggie omelet makes a nutritious, quick dish for any mealtime. Hard-boiled eggs make wonderful snacks, alone or in green salads.)
- Sugar-free instant bean soup mixes, such as Fantastic Foods black bean or refried bean flakes

* Both beans and quinoa need to be checked for small stones and rinsed thoroughly before cooking. Quinoa is ready to cook when the rinse water runs clear.

Just because a food has a reputation for healthfulness, or a label suggesting that it's good for you, doesn't mean it's low in sugar (or, for that matter, low in other undesirable ingredients or properties). Check labels carefully, and stick to the "one-ingredient rule"; look for fresh vegetables instead of packaged; choose plain yogurt or oatmeal and add your own flavorings if you want them (but not dates, honey, etc.).

Foods to toss:

Of course, if the sugar content on any of these items is low, then you can keep it.

- Soy, almond, or rice milk
- Yogurt, except for unsweetened
- Cereal (except for slow-cooking oatmeal or porridge, quinoa flakes, or unsweetened kasha)
- Tomato sauce
- Energy/protein bars
- Milk
- Alcohol

KITCHEN TOOLS AND EQUIPMENT

Depending on your personal meal-preparation style—that is, whether you're a slavish follower of recipes or the type who creates your own as you go along—you'll want to make sure your kitchen contains at least some of the following:

- Measuring cup (unless you are the second kind of cook)
- Vegetable peeler (very useful for making Mock Pasta Ribbons, page 103)
- Large skillet or frying pan (Stainless steel or copper is the most highly recommended kind.)

- Stockpot for cooking things like quinoa
- Glass baking dish
- Whisk for omelets (Though you can use a fork, if you prefer.)
- Good-size bowl for mixing
- Salad bowl
- Sharp knife for dicing vegetables
- Garlic press
- Strainer
- Spatula for turning omelets
- Wooden spoon
- Reusable plastic containers, so you can take salads and other meals to work
- Cutting board (Marble can be cleaned fairly easily, though it is heavy; unlike wood or plastic, it tends not to retain substances on its surface.)
- Pressure cooker for preparing dried beans relatively quickly without the bother of soaking them overnight (optional)

Note: Glass and stainless steel are on the safer side of the cooking-materials spectrum and are relatively easy to clean. They also tend not to discolor.

THE POWER OF PRESENTATION

The better a dish looks, the more we'll want to eat it. Try to give meals as much visual appeal as you can, especially if you're trying to help your family adjust to a new way of eating. That doesn't mean that you need to present each plate with the panache of a Paris pastry chef, but it does mean that you hold the power to influence how enticing your preparations appear.

For example, instead of plopping your mock pasta ribbons or soba noodles onto a dish, take an extra moment (for that is all it will take) to twirl them pleasingly around a fork, and then release onto the serving platter or individual plate. Sprinkle on a teaspoon or two of toasted sesame seeds, perhaps some coarsely ground black pepper. Voilà! A meal fit for a Parisian palate, but just as pleasing to an American one.

Quinoa, in particular, presses nicely into mounds or fancy molded shapes. That's not to say you need to go all Martha Stewart every time—but for company or especially finicky family members, the little extra effort might prove worth it.

Other healthful, sugar-free elements that also add visual appeal include:

- Thinly sliced red bell pepper
- Broccoli florets and leaves
- Cherry tomatoes, especially halved
- White or black pepper
- Sesame seeds (which come in white and black varieties; try using different colors for contrast)

You might find it's kind of fun to dress up your meals—and the compliments you receive will probably be fun to hear as well.

SPECIAL DIETARY CONSIDERATIONS

If you have more than one dietary need—that is, if you want to cleanse your body of sugar, but are also a vegetarian, are watching sodium, have allergies, or need to eat kosher or halal meals—you should be able to adapt any of these recipes to your specific needs or wants. Vegetarians should be able to use or adapt most of these recipes with little difficulty. Tofu or other proteins can easily replace the protein found in meats or fish. Hummus, egg, avocado, Parmesan or feta cheese, fruit or yogurt snacks can, in most cases, replace nuts.

The recipes in this book do not contain added salt. The sodium in virtually all of these recipes can be omitted or limited with little loss of flavor or texture. (Some of the soy or prepackaged recipe ingredients may be high in sodium, however. You should be able to substitute other detox recipes for these.) Almost all of these recipes are also naturally gluten-free.

And if you don't care for a particular vegetable, for instance? Relax. In most cases, you can substitute one detox-diet-permissible vegetable for another.

RESTAURANTS, CELEBRATIONS, AND EVENTS

Depending on how often you eat out (or find yourself at weddings, bar mitzvahs, and the like) and how dedicated you want to be, you may have no shortage of challenges to navigate while on sugar detox.

Your best bet will usually be to call ahead. Explain to the powers that be, "I need a sugar-free entrée—and, ideally, a sugar-free choice of appetizer and dessert," or something like that. (It's good to have choices.) Good restaurants and facilities will be only too happy to accommodate. If you find yourself on the wrong end of a choice ("Well, everything comes into the kitchen already made," to cite one example), then it's best to strategize. Ask for recommendations for the lowest-sugar offering or bring your own. Or say that you need a sugar-restricted, diabetic-safe meal. That should frighten most kitchens into cooperation.

If telling a white lie isn't your style (and frankly, we're not crazy about it)—or if you haven't called ahead and made arrangements—you can ask for "no added sugar." In Asian restaurants, you can sometimes ask for "kitchen rice." Yes, many restaurants add sugar even to ordinary items such as rice. Why do you think California rolls taste so good? Most restaurant and hotel kitchens can prepare fruit plates on request. If everyone else at the table is ordering dessert or it is included in your meal, the fresh fruit plate might represent a decent choice.

Remember to ask, too, about milk, especially condensed milk, in soups, sauces, and gravies. Eating out can be a huge challenge for sugar detoxers (although the recent popularity of the diet may be changing that somewhat). If at all possible, save eating out for special occasions. Neighborhood takeout may be OK—you'll need to investigate this on your own—but most chain restaurants pour inordinate amounts of sugar (and salt and often fat) into their products to make them delicious. Beware. If nothing else, ask for olive oil and fresh lemon, or bring your own, for your green salad.

INFORMAL OUTINGS

If you're planning to spend an afternoon or evening at the ballpark, for example, you might want to tote your own snacks. A bag or two of cut-up green apples, red bell pepper slices, nuts, or washed strawberries can feed your need for snacks without spoiling your diet or forcing you to go hungry. If the evening's entertainment is a long opera, you're on your own!

TRAVEL

If you're traveling for a day or so, you might be wise to take along your own healthful snacks. Bell pepper slices, nuts, hard-boiled eggs, even small containers of dishes such as Spaghetti Squash Sauté (page 104) or Quinoa Vegetable Sauté (page 108) usually travel fairly well. If you plan to be on the road for a few days or more, you might want to choose accommodations with refrigerators or kitchenettes, or observe the previous tips from "Restaurants, Celebrations and Events."

WHEN YOU'RE THE "COMPANY"

If invited to another person's home, you want to be polite—but you also want to keep your resolve intact. Try not to demand too much extra attention from your host.

Consider the following:

- Choosing carefully from the items offered
- Taking small portions of everything (or at least, everything that appeals to you)
- Making this outing your occasional "splurge"
- Skipping it
- Asking for permission to bring your own dish (with enough to share, naturally), to minimize the discomfort others may feel if you're sitting at the table with them, but not eating.

You may have to decide, of course, whether you want to discuss your dietary behavior and philosophy with others, including your host. Needless to say, it's up to you. If your comfort level is high, or you're feeling evangelical, go for it! No reason to keep these kinds of things a secret. Sugar isn't good for anyone else, either. On the other hand, if you would rather keep your preferences and food habits to yourself, that's fine, too. It doesn't have to be anybody else's business unless you want it to be.

THE IMPORTANCE OF EXERCISE

What you eat every day has a tremendous effect on your overall health. Of course, as you no doubt know, exercise holds great importance as well. For most people, a half-hour walk each day can go a long way—so to speak—in helping you attain and maintain your best health. Talk to your doctor to help determine which kinds of exercise and how much might be right for you.

Exercise doesn't have to be a boring or miserable chore. Dancing is exercise. So is roller-skating. So are horseback riding and zip-lining and canoeing. The trick is to exercise consistently, properly, and safely (which is where your doctor comes in). Experiment until you find an activity you like and can stick to.

ORGANICS: TO BUY OR NOT TO BUY?

Organic produce is grown without most synthetic pesticides, chemical fertilizers, irradiation, and additives. Organic foods also do not contain genetically modified organisms, or GMOs. Therefore, organic food is often viewed as beneficial to one's health (at least, not as harmful as conventional foods).

To some, however, organic food is unnecessarily expensive. It is sometimes said that consumers are paying more for cachet than nutritional value. Do a little research and draw your own conclusions.

If you do want to go organic, but are daunted by the prices, these quick tips might help:

- Check your local supermarket rather than depending on stores that carry exclusively organic products.
- Farmers' markets often offer high-quality (though not necessarily organic) produce, exotic new veggies, and generally fresh, flavorful, colorful choices—sometimes, though not always, at a bargain. One added benefit: You can talk directly with the farmers about their practices.
- Choose fruits and vegetables in season. Watch for the lowest prices. Melon and berries, for instance, are usually least expensive in summer, when they are in large supply. This applies to organic as well as conventional produce. Although fresh is usually best, you can buy passable frozen fruits and veggies. Check labels to make sure you're getting only the produce, and not added sugar—or for that matter, salt.

Are you familiar with the "Dirty Dozen" (and "Clean Fifteen") lists? Since organic produce and other products can be expensive, the Environmental Working Group releases an annual list of the twelve biggest offenders (and the fifteen cleanest), in terms of pesticides and other contaminants, to help consumers make wholesome choices when shopping. Check the site (www.ewg.org) often for guidance on clean and healthful produce.

FISH: FARMED VS. WILD

Although there are exceptions, wild fish—particularly salmon—is often considered the better nutritional value. Wild salmon swims considerable lengths, making it extra lean (imagine a flabby couch-potato salmon, if such a thing existed!). However, that is not to say that all wild salmon is always better than all farmed fish. Not at all. Some farmed fish is very high in quality. Wild-caught fish are subject to environmental contaminants, for one thing (an issue of even greater concern since the Fukushima disaster in 2011). So what should you do? Educate yourself as much as you can. One good source is the National Cooperative Grocers Association (www.ncga.org; for information about fish specifically, visit NCGA's page on the topic: www.ncga.coop/newsroom/fish).

READING LABELS

Avoiding sugar isn't always easy. One reason for that is product labeling.

Labeling laws state that package ingredients be listed according to their prevalence; that is, ingredients are listed from highest concentration to lowest. So if the product contains 80 percent water, "water" is the first item you'll see on the label. If it contains a pinch of pepper, you'll see that listed at the very end (probably as "spices," as most companies don't want their competitors to know exactly what they contain and in which proportions). Today, most companies know that listing "sugar" as the primary ingredient won't make them look good to consumers—particularly those shopping for their young kids. So they use a few different kinds of sugar in each product. Therefore, a label might read, for instance: "flour, cane sugar, fructose, whey, honey ..." See that? Three different kinds of sugar you might have missed if you were in a hurry, confused (understandable, given all the different names for one thing), or simply unable to read the small print.

The solution? Well, there's one rather simple answer, as you read earlier in this chapter: the one-ingredient food! Fresh vegetables, fruits, grain substitutes, eggs, and beans are great examples.

What does *sugar-free* mean? By *sugar-free*, some companies and cookbooks really mean "but it does contain honey ... that's not the same thing, right?" Wrong. Read labels. Sugar-free should mean devoid of any added sweeteners, whether barley malt, fructose, honey, corn syrup, evaporated cane juice, and so on.

THINGS TO DISCUSS WITH YOUR DOCTOR

Of course, you don't expect cutting out sugar to turn out to be a *bad* thing. But there are some things you might want to discuss with your doctor in terms of your diet, general health, and new eating plan.

For instance, in cutting sugar out of your diet, are you planning to add more salt? That could be dangerous. Same with fats. Increasing your intake of nuts, for example, could end up raising your salt and fat consumption and your overall weight. (This is less likely to happen if you consume them as directed, however.)

If you have diabetes or know that you are at risk for the disease, make sure to talk with your doctor before beginning any new diet plan, even a low- or no-sugar one such as this.

Especially if you are a vegetarian, talk with your doctor about whether a plant-based diet will provide you with enough protein. If not, he or she might want to recommend one or more supplements.

Athletes, new mothers, and women who are pregnant or would like to be will have special concerns to address with their doctors, of course.

Your doctor may want to start with a blood test to determine whether you have or are at risk for high blood sugar or diabetes. They may want to test your cholesterol, blood pressure, or any number of things. Let them know that you are interested in "detoxing" from sugar, and about any vitamins or supplements that you already take or may wish to take.

TEN TIPS FOR A SUCCESSFUL SUGAR DETOX

1. Your most powerful tool is your mind. Use it wisely. Remind yourself often that you're getting your body into tip-top shape. Inhale slowly and smile on the exhale. Now do it again!
2. Remember that the first three to five days are the hardest. The less sugar you have in your body, the less you'll crave it.
3. Prepare as much food as possible in advance so that when hunger strikes, you can meet it with good nutrition. Obviously, don't keep so much food on hand that it tempts you unduly or spoils before you can eat it. If you find it hard to cook food without eating the results of your labor immediately, don't spend the whole day cooking!
4. Do stuff. This might be a great time to start another new project. Keep your mind, and ideally your hands, busy with something productive.

5. Be patient with yourself. If you "fall off the wagon," climb right back on (and don't wait till tomorrow, either). Don't let your inner voice say cruel or negative things. Replace those sentiments with "I can do this!" and the knowledge that you will look and feel better with less (or no) sugar in your system.

6. Avoid temptation. You know where it lurks. Whether in the office coffee cart, Monday morning meeting, rail station kiosk, or snack foods aisle at the grocery store—run in the other direction.

7. Get help. Letting your friends, family, and workmates know that you're embarking on a new eating plan will make you accountable. If you find your willpower flagging, enlist help from a friend. If you and at least one friend can start on this diet together, so much the better.

8. Begin each day with a large and satisfying breakfast. This will help you keep cravings at bay immediately—and also give you the energy you need to start your day!

9. Don't sweat the small stuff! If you need to substitute a nut-free, vegetarian, kosher, or halal entrée for one of the meat dishes recommended on your diet plan, feel free to do so. Success—not slavish devotion to rules that might not be right for you—is your ultimate goal.

10. Get sufficient exercise. (See the earlier sections "The Importance of Exercise" and "Things to Discuss with Your Doctor.")

CHAPTER 3

Sugar Detox Meal Plans

This book features two sugar detox meal plans: a 3-day plan and a more gradual 21-day plan.

Which one is right for you? This, of course, is a question that only you can answer. Do you want to see results immediately? Do you feel enthusiastic? Do you long to just feel better already or change your lifestyle for the better, quickly? Are you unafraid of jumping in? Sounds as if you want the three-day plan.

Would you prefer to take a more gradual approach? Are you trying to bring other family members along with you? Do you believe in slow, steady changes for lifelong good habits? For that, you might prefer a gradual detox.

A gradual plan is not extreme and holds the added advantage of being a plan you can live with over the long term. The quick plan will help you get sugar out of your system that much faster. Or you might decide to start with the three-day plan, but graduate immediately to the maximum number of foods allowable on the detox diet. That's fine, too. Remember, it's all good—as long as it's sugar-free!

Still relying on three square meals a day? That's fine—but there's no reason to stick to that. Many people have found that five, or even six, mini-meals throughout the day regulate blood sugar and weight, and minimize cravings. At the very least, please give up the idea of eating your biggest meal at night, when you least need the calories and energy it provides.

SOME THINGS TO KEEP IN MIND

The recipes in this book range from easy to slightly challenging, to accommodate all levels of chefs, from uneasy in the kitchen to unabashedly adventurous. Some will yield "family size" portions; others are intended for one. The majority are simple, so that just about anyone can prepare them easily and enjoy them immediately.

A quick caveat: When cutting out sugar, take care not to substitute other unhealthful ingredients such as salt or fat. For flavor and extra appeal, use spices. Most are perfectly fine, especially in moderation.

Know, too, that it is important to consume a varied, balanced diet. **It is not recommended that you continue on the strict three-day detox meal plan beyond three days.** By all means, however, continue to avoid added sugar. (See "Things to Discuss with Your Doctor" in Chapter 2.) In addition, make yourself aware of the ingredients in your food and about nutrition in general. Nothing will serve you better.

If work or family responsibilities keep you too busy to do much cooking, you might want to take advantage of ready-roasted turkey and chicken, canned beans, and so on. You should still be able to eat fresh fruits or throw together salads to take to work the next day. As you have no doubt discovered, cooking over the weekend helps, too.

A word about portions: How much to eat will depend on why you want to detox from sugar—to combat mood swings, yeast infections, or an overall dependence, or to lose weight? Generally speaking, you should not feel hungry on the Sugar Detox Diet. Most of the recipes in this book will not cause weight gain.

If you're concerned about calories, reduce your intake of avocados, nuts, nut butters, and cheese, and keep an eye on the amount of milk and sweet fruits you consume (see "Things to Discuss with Your Doctor" in Chapter 2). Green apples, bell peppers, egg whites, and virtually all green vegetables can be enjoyed at any time.

Finally, remember the golden rule for any diet plan: Eat when you're hungry. Don't eat when you're not.

BREAKFAST: THE MOST IMPORTANT MEAL OF THE DAY

Have you ever heard it said that you should eat breakfast like a king (or queen), lunch like a prince (or princess), and dinner like a pauper? Consuming most of your protein and calories at the beginning of your day will give you the energy you need to do your work and get adequate exercise—and hopefully prepare more nutritious meals in the bargain!

This plan includes a few light breakfasts for those who can't tolerate a lot of food first thing—but we recommend perhaps a light snack first, if this is the case for you, and a bigger breakfast later in the morning. That is, simply switch the order of your breakfast and mid-morning snack.

Salmon for breakfast? Don't knock it! In Japan, lots of people start their day with high-protein fish. Think about reinventing your ideas of breakfast, lunch, and dinner.

BEVERAGES: SOME DOS AND DON'TS

Must all beverages have distinct flavors? By no means! Water is plain and almost perfect. Cucumber slices or lemon or lime wedges can jazz it up. So can serving it ice-cold, although some believe it's more healthful to drink it at room temperature. If you need something sweet to flavor your tea, you might want to try a touch of stevia. But keep in mind, as you read in Chapter 1, that its use is still relatively new in this country. There even are chocolate-flavored teas!

Soft drinks have no place in a healthful diet. Cola, pop, soda, soda pop … whatever you call it, the romance must end, immediately and forever. Painful though it may be, if you want to stay sugar- and artificial sweetener–free, you need to say, "Sweet Fanny Adams, buh-bye!"

Proper hydration is important to good health. Make sure to drink adequate amounts of water, especially if you're used to downing sodas, fruit juice, or other less-than-healthful beverages. Sixty-four ounces of water a day is the standard recommendation. Let thirst be your guide, but don't go too far in either direction. Coffee is not forbidden, but please do consider tea, especially green or white tea; the health benefits of tea are well documented. If you can't stand the plainness of unflavored water, by all means add a slice of lime, a squeeze of lemon juice, or a slice of cucumber, or keep your water well-chilled.

THREE-DAY DETOX

Because of sugar's addictive properties, the first three days will be the hardest. If you can get past this period in which your cravings will be at their strongest, you'll have won more than half of the battle. Cravings may persist, but they'll get weaker as your time away from sugar continues. The following plan will help provide strong weaponry for the fight!

Detoxing "cold turkey" will get you looking and feeling better that much faster. (Speaking of which, cold cooked turkey, provided there's no glaze, sauce, or stuffing, should be fine to eat!) There's no margin of error—follow this plan exactly and you'll be eating the sugar-free way.

Remember, though, that the detox diet is infinitely flexible, too. If you need to substitute one day's meals or snacks for another, go for it. You should derive equal nutritional and detox benefits.

To derive more value from the detox diet, eat small amounts of protein throughout the day—at least every four hours—and drink plenty of water (spring water is especially recommended for its purity).

You need variety—excluding sugar, of course—in your diet. Treat these meal plans as guidelines. For best results, take a look at the recipes in the other sections, too. If you want to continue "sugar-free," avoid the healthful but sugary fruits and vegetables noted earlier in the book.

A few more tricks:

- Try to use well-loved plates and dishes, which can impart a feeling of comfort.
- Take the time to eat slowly and carefully, and enjoy your food. Smile. Sigh contentedly. Think sincerely about how comforting, filling, and delicious your food looks. It may sound kooky, but it often pays to enlist your mind to help your body.
- If you feel deprived or are craving sugar, try a snack such as spiced nuts, get busy cooking a new recipe, or turn to the crave-busting tips listed earlier in this book.
- Sadly, milk and other dairy products contain naturally occurring sugars (and sometimes added sweetener)—so three-day detoxers are asked to forgo dairy products during the initial detox period. If you want to add them back in judiciously later, you may do so. Please talk with your health care provider about whether, and in what amounts, dairy products should be included in your overall diet.

And finally, keep in mind:

- Labels (make sure to read them)
- Hidden sugar (such as you find in dates, corn, parsnips, watermelon, sweet potatoes, etc.)

An old dieting trick Slice snacks into small strips. That way, you'll be forced to eat them slowly, giving that old satiety signal plenty of time to reach your brain.

DAY 1

BREAKFAST:

SLOW-COOKED PORRIDGE OR OATMEAL

FRESH BLUEBERRIES*

FRESH STRAWBERRIES*

GROUND CINNAMON, IF DESIRED

GREEN TEA

Prepare porridge according to package directions. Pour into a bowl and top with blueberries and sliced strawberries. Add cinnamon if desired.

* You may substitute frozen berries, if necessary. Always wash fresh produce before using.

MID-MORNING SNACK:

ALMONDS, RAW OR DRY ROASTED (CHECK PACKAGE LABEL FOR ANY HIDDEN SWEETENERS)—NO MORE THAN 10 (THEY'RE FATTENING!)

LUNCH:

BABY SPINACH AND ARUGULA SALAD, DRESSED WITH 1 TABLESPOON OLIVE OIL AND FRESH-SQUEEZED LEMON JUICE

QUINOA VEGETABLE SAUTÉ (PAGE 108)

AFTERNOON SNACK:

½ AVOCADO OR ½ CUP GUACAMOLE (PAGE 83)

DINNER:

SALMON TERIYAKI† (PAGE 116)

KASHA

WILTED SPINACH, STEAMED ASPARAGUS, OR STEAMED BROCCOLI, DRESSED WITH FRESHLY SQUEEZED LEMON AND DRIZZLED WITH OLIVE OIL

† You can substitute chicken or tofu. Make sure to cook thoroughly.

DESSERT:

SLICED GREEN APPLE WITH CINNAMON (CONSUME AS IS IF YOU LIKE A TANGY CRUNCH; WARM IN OVEN TO BRING OUT THE APPLE'S NATURAL SWEETNESS FOR SOMETHING MORE LIKE AN APPLE PIE)

DAY 2

BREAKFAST:

VEGGIE OMELET MADE FROM 3 EGGS, BUT ONLY ONE OF THE YOLKS (SEE
   SUPER SUPPER OMELET, PAGE 112, OR CREATE YOUR OWN)
CANTALOUPE WEDGE, ⅓ CUP BLUEBERRIES OR SLICED STRAWBERRIES,
   OR BOTH
GREEN TEA

MID-MORNING SNACK:

⅓ CUP WARMED EDAMAME BEANS

LUNCH:

WHOLE CAN OR POUCH OF TUNA, OR A FRESH TUNA STEAK, ABOUT
   ⅓ POUND, WITH FRESH LEMON JUICE
GREEN SALAD MADE WITH ROMAINE LETTUCE, PARSLEY, RED
   BELL PEPPER STRIPS, CUCUMBER, OR YOUR CHOICE OF GREEN
   VEGETABLES, DRESSED WITH 1 TABLESPOON OLIVE OIL AND FRESH
   LEMON JUICE
1 CUP STEAMED BROCCOLI, ALSO DRESSED WITH FRESH LEMON JUICE
   AND 1 TABLESPOON OR LESS OF OLIVE OIL AND FRESHLY GROUND
   PEPPER, IF DESIRED

AFTERNOON SNACK:

SLICED MIXED BELL PEPPERS WITH LEMONY HUMMUS (PAGE 90)

DINNER:

LEAN ROASTED CHICKEN SLICES
ROASTED BRUSSELS (PAGE 128)
MOCK POTATOES (PAGE 132)

DESSERT:

PEAR

DAY 3

BREAKFAST:

BREAKFAST SALMON (PAGE 75) WITH 1 CUP PLAIN QUINOA

CANTALOUPE, BERRIES, OR BOTH, IF DESIRED

MID-MORNING SNACK:

SLICED HARD-BOILED EGG WITH BOK CHOI; FLAVOR WITH A DRIZZLE OF
OLIVE OIL, LEMON JUICE, AND PEPPER, IF YOU WISH

LUNCH:

SLICES OF LEAN CHICKEN ATOP A LARGE GREEN SALAD

STEAMED BROCCOLI, SPINACH, OR ASPARAGUS

AFTERNOON SNACK:

1 CUP LEMONY HUMMUS (PAGE 90) WITH CELERY STICKS, OR PLAIN
4 OLIVES, BLACK OR GREEN, OR ½ CUP GUACAMOLE (PAGE 83)

DINNER:

SPAGHETTI SQUASH SAUTÉ (PAGE 104)

GREEN SALAD

DESSERT:

BAKED APPLE (PAGE 135)

According to the Poland Spring Water company, the average 12-ounce sugar-sweetened beverage contains about 10 teaspoons of sugar or the equivalent. Cut out one of those sugary drinks a day and lose a whopping 3,650 teaspoons of sugar over the course of one year. Drink mostly water only and you can easily lose an additional . . . we can't count that high!

GRADUAL DETOX (21 DAYS)

Gradually shedding your dependence on sugar can make a new man or woman of you. As you replace old habits with new healthful ones, you'll find that not only do you look and feel so much better, but also that your new behaviors are "sticking." That's the beauty of making small changes over time.

A few tips to help you enjoy successful moderation:

- Remember the "first few bites" rule: taste, then toss. (Nobody likes to waste food, of course. But you don't want to treat yourself like a human garbage pail, either—or subject others to the same health risks. Shampoo your hair with unwanted egg yolks, or feed them to your dog or cat. Use that brown sugar with your favorite cream cleanser to make an economical facial scrub.) On the other hand, bear in mind the words of exercise guru Denise Austin: "A sliver leads to a slab, and a slab leads to a slob." If you know you won't stop eating until the entire carton of ice cream is just a sickly sweet memory, don't get started. In the words of another famously thin woman, "Just say no."

- A little goes a long way. Instead of wine, for instance, choose a spritzer. That way, you still get to enjoy a little wine, but you've cut the sugar and alcohol content significantly—assuming you stick to just one or two glasses. (For gradual detoxers, the occasional glass of red wine should be OK—provided you do not have a problem with alcohol or alcoholism and are not underage.) Similarly, if you find yourself craving cheese or sour cream, add just a touch to your omelet or mock pasta. You probably won't need a whole lot in order to feel satisfied.

- Reward yourself—a little. Enjoy some ice cream or cake on your birthday, for instance (unless the taste of sugar weakens your resolve against more; if that's true for you, you might want to employ the full-on detox plan).

- Gradual detoxers may use fruit and dairy products, so long as they don't go overboard. A little sweet fruit can be your friend. Strawberries and blueberries are not only sweet; they are also high in antioxidants, as you may know. An added benefit? Strawberries, blueberries, and also cantaloupe can impart a healthful glow to your skin. If you wish, you can freeze these sweet fruits (or a few grapes) to bring out their natural sweetness. (Also see recipe for Baked Apple, page 135.)

- Make sure to drink plenty of water. Antioxidant-rich green or white tea is also recommended, especially at breakfast time.

As with the three-day detox, you may substitute one meal or snack for another. Just make sure you're getting sufficient protein and vegetables each day. A few tips for easier digestion:

- Especially at first, while you're getting used to this new way of eating, choose cooked vegetables over raw. If you do plan to eat raw veggies, chop them well first.

- Plain quinoa tends to be mild on the stomach.

- Peppermint or other stomach-soothing teas can be helpful.

The meal plans on the following pages are designed for maximum flexibility. Above all, please keep in mind that they are only guidelines. As you read earlier in this book, it's important that you talk with your doctor before embarking on any new diet.

DAY 1

BREAKFAST:

SUPER SUPPER OMELET (PAGE 112)

CANTALOUPE WEDGE

½ CUP FRESH STRAWBERRIES OR BLUEBERRIES

GREEN TEA

MID-MORNING SNACK:

RED BELL PEPPER SLICES (EAT AS MANY AS YOU WANT, BUT BEAR IN
MIND THAT TOO MANY FRUITS OR VEGGIES AT ONCE CAN PLAY HAVOC
WITH YOUR DIGESTION; SEE THE DIGESTION TIPS ON PAGE 37)

LUNCH:

QUINOA VEGETABLE SAUTÉ (PAGE 108)

BABY SPINACH AND ARUGULA SALAD, DRESSED WITH 1 TABLESPOON
OLIVE OIL, FRESHLY SQUEEZED LEMON JUICE, AND PEPPER,
IF DESIRED

AFTERNOON SNACK:

1 CUP UNSWEETENED YOGURT WITH UP TO 1 TABLESPOON GROUND
CINNAMON

DINNER:

SALMON TERIYAKI (PAGE 116)

STEAMED BROCCOLI, SPINACH, OR ASPARAGUS

MOCK POTATOES (PAGE 132)

EVENING SNACK:

GUACAMOLE (PAGE 83)

DAY 2

BREAKFAST:

SUPER SUPPER OMELET (PAGE 112)

GREEN TEA

MID-MORNING SNACK:

½ GRAPEFRUIT (OR A WHOLE ONE IF YOU'RE ESPECIALLY HUNGRY)

LUNCH:

LENTIL SOUP (PAGE 93)

PARMA CRISPS (PAGE 88)

AFTERNOON SNACK:

10 ROASTED UNSALTED ALMONDS OR CASHEWS

DINNER:

SIMPLE ROASTED CHICKEN (PAGE 120)

STEAMED BROCCOLI, SPINACH, OR ASPARAGUS

MOCK PASTA RIBBONS (PAGE 103)

DESSERT:

BAKED APPLE (PAGE 135) OR YOGURT SUPREME (PAGE 66)

DAY 3

BREAKFAST:

SLOW-COOKED OATMEAL OR PORRIDGE

½ CUP SLICED BERRIES

MILK OR MILK SUBSTITUTE

GREEN TEA

MID-MORNING SNACK:

¼ CUP SUNFLOWER SEEDS

LUNCH:

LEAN TURKEY BURGER

TOMATO SLICES

ROMAINE LETTUCE WITH PARSLEY, DRESSED WITH 1 TABLESPOON OLIVE
    OIL AND FRESH LEMON JUICE

MOCK POTATOES (PAGE 132)

AFTERNOON SNACK:

½ CUP LEMONY HUMMUS (PAGE 90) WITH ½ RED BELL PEPPER, SLICED

DINNER:

CHELSEA CHICKEN SOUP (PAGE 94)

EVENING SNACK:

HARD-BOILED EGG

DAY 4

BREAKFAST:

UNSWEETENED YOGURT WITH SLICED GREEN APPLES AND SLIVERED
ALMONDS

GREEN TEA

MID-MORNING SNACK:

5 ALMOND CRACKERS (PAGE 89)

PEAR

LUNCH:

BOWL OF INSTANT BLACK OR REFRIED BEAN SOUP, SUCH AS FANTASTIC
FOODS BRAND, WITH A DOLLOP OF PLAIN, UNSWEETENED YOGURT
OR SHREDDED CHEESE AND FRESH PARSLEY, IF DESIRED

GREEN SALAD

AFTERNOON SNACK:

4 OR 5 OLIVES

DINNER:

SZECHUAN TOFU (PAGE 114)

PEAR & POM SALAD (PAGE 95)

DESSERT:

BAKED APPLE (PAGE 135)

DAY 5

BREAKFAST:

TWO EGGS, ANY STYLE

2 SLICES TURKEY BACON OR TURKEY SAUSAGE PATTIES (PAGE 76)

GREEN TEA

MID-MORNING SNACK:

PEACH NUT PARFAIT (PAGE 65)

LUNCH:

TOFU SALAD (PAGE 100)

½ RED BELL PEPPER, SLICED

AFTERNOON SNACK:

GREEN APPLE WITH 1 TABLESPOON ALMOND BUTTER

DINNER:

MOCK BREADED EGGPLANT (PAGE 105)

PLAIN QUINOA

EVENING SNACK:

TEN ALMONDS OR OTHER NUTS

DAY 6

BREAKFAST:

SUPER SUPPER OMELET (PAGE 112)

½ CUP BERRIES

GREEN TEA

MID-MORNING SNACK:

WARMED EDAMAME BEANS

LUNCH:

GRILLED TUNA

STEAMED BROCCOLI

TOMATO SLICES

AFTERNOON SNACK:

PEACH

DINNER:

HOMEMADE FALAFEL (PAGE 113) WITH SLICED TOMATOES, CUCUMBERS, AND ROMAINE LETTUCE

PLAIN QUINOA

DESSERT:

SLICED APPLE WITH 1 TABLESPOON ALMOND BUTTER

DAY 7

BREAKFAST:

AUTHENTIC PORRIDGE (PAGE 62)

½ CUP MILK OR MILK SUBSTITUTE

½ CUP BERRIES OF YOUR CHOICE

MID-MORNING SNACK:

KALE CHIPS (PAGE 81)

LUNCH:

SOBA STIR-FRY (PAGE 107)

ROMAINE, PARSLEY, AND BOK CHOI SALAD WITH 1 TABLESPOON OIL-AND-
VINEGAR DRESSING

AFTERNOON SNACK:

AVOCADO SLICES (½ OR WHOLE AVOCADO)

DINNER:

LEMON-LIME CHICKEN

GRILLED ASPARAGUS (PAGE 124) OR ROASTED BRUSSELS (PAGE 128)

DESSERT:

COTTAGE CHEESE WITH CINNAMON

DAY 8

BREAKFAST:

BREAKFAST EGG SALAD (PAGE 68)

RED PEPPER OR CUCUMBER SLICES

MID-MORNING SNACK:

PEAR

LUNCH:

SALMON BURGER

SLICED TOMATO

GREEN SALAD OF ROMAINE LETTUCE, FRESH PARSLEY, CUCUMBER, AND
   PEPPERS; BOILED EGG OR GARBANZO BEANS, IF DESIRED

AFTERNOON SNACK:

EASY AVOCADO-TURKEY ROLLS (PAGE 84)

DINNER:

SPAGHETTI SQUASH SAUTÉ

GREEN SALAD

DESSERT:

BROILED GRAPEFRUIT (PAGE 78)

DAY 9

BREAKFAST:

YOGURT SUPREME (PAGE 66)

GREEN TEA

MID-MORNING SNACK:

HARD-BOILED EGG

LUNCH:

SUPER SUPPER SALAD (PAGE 96); OMIT EGG IF YOU NEED TO LIMIT YOUR
 CONSUMPTION. FEEL FREE TO ADD OR SUBSTITUTE GRILLED
 CHICKEN STRIPS.

PARMA CRISPS (PAGE 88)

AFTERNOON SNACK:

CRUDITÉ OF BROCCOLI, CAULIFLOWER, ZUCCHINI, WITH 1 TABLESPOON
 OLIVE OIL AND FRESHLY SQUEEZED LEMON JUICE FOR DIPPING

DINNER:

FISH KEBABS (PAGE 115)

QUINOA

STEAMED BROCCOLI, ASPARAGUS, SPINACH, OR BRUSSELS SPROUTS
 WITH 1 OR 2 TABLESPOONS OLIVE OIL, FRESHLY SQUEEZED LEMON
 JUICE, AND FRESHLY GROUND BLACK PEPPER TO TASTE

EVENING SNACK:

5–10 ALMONDS OR HAZELNUTS

DAY 10

BREAKFAST:

BREAKFAST SALMON (PAGE 75)

STEAMED BROCCOLI WITH FRESH LEMON JUICE

MID-MORNING SNACK:

APPLE AND PEAR SLICES WITH 1 TABLESPOON PEANUT BUTTER

LUNCH:

LENTIL SOUP (PAGE 93)

AFTERNOON SNACK:

WATERCRESS SALAD WITH RED AND YELLOW BELL PEPPER STRIPS,
    1 TABLESPOON OLIVE OIL, FRESH LEMON JUICE

DINNER:

SIMPLE ROASTED CHICKEN (PAGE 120)

PLAIN QUINOA

SAUTEED SPINACH

EVENING SNACK:

TOASTED SOY NUTS

DAY 11

BREAKFAST:

YOGURT SUPREME (PAGE 67)

CANTALOUPE OR HONEYDEW WEDGE

MID-MORNING SNACK:

¼ CUP SUNFLOWER SEEDS

LUNCH:

SALAD SAUTÉ (PAGE 97)

MOCK PASTA RIBBONS (PAGE 103) OR AVOCADO SLICES

AFTERNOON SNACK:

SLICED GREEN APPLE WITH CINNAMON AND ¼ CUP SLIVERED ALMONDS

DINNER:

GRILLED TROUT

SESAME ZUCCHINI (PAGE 126)

MOCK POTATOES (PAGE 132)

DESSERT:

5 CHOCOLATE-DIPPED STRAWBERRIES (PAGE 137)

DAY 12

BREAKFAST:

LOW-CARB KASHA VARNISHKAS (PAGE 63)

8 OUNCES SKIM OR LOW-FAT MILK

MID-MORNING SNACK:

½ CUP COTTAGE CHEESE

SLICED GREEN APPLE

LUNCH:

CLAM CHOWDER

PARMA CRISPS (PAGE 88)

AFTERNOON SNACK:

GUACAMOLE (PAGE 83)

TOMATO SLICES

DINNER:

GRILLED SALMON

WILTED SPINACH

KASHA

DESSERT:

PEACH NUT PARFAIT (PAGE 65)

DAY 13

BREAKFAST:

LEFTOVER GRILLED OR BROILED SALMON

THREE BEAN SALAD

MID-MORNING SNACK:

TOASTED PUMPKIN SEEDS (PAGE 85)

LUNCH:

SMALL TUNA STEAK OR INDIVIDUAL CAN OR POUCH

SOBA NOODLES

RED BELL PEPPER SLICES AND BROCCOLI FLORETS

AFTERNOON SNACK:

5 MACADAMIA NUTS

DINNER:

COLD QUINOA SALAD (PAGE 98)

DESSERT:

GREEN APPLE SLICES WITH CINNAMON

DAY 14

BREAKFAST:

VEGGIE OMELET WITH 2 SLICES TURKEY BACON

MID-MORNING SNACK:

CANTALOUPE WEDGE

STRAWBERRIES OR BLUEBERRIES

LUNCH:

BROILED HALIBUT

ROASTED BRUSSELS (PAGE 128)

MOCK PASTA RIBBONS (PAGE 103)

AFTERNOON SNACK:

BROILED GRAPEFRUIT (PAGE 78)

DINNER:

RED LENTIL SALAD (PAGE 99)

EVENING SNACK:

¼ CUP ROASTED CASHEWS

DAY 15

BREAKFAST:

SLOW-COOKED OATMEAL

BERRIES

MILK

MID-MORNING SNACK:

PEACH NUT PARFAIT (PAGE 65)

LUNCH:

STEAMED EDAMAME BEANS

COLD QUINOA SALAD (PAGE 98)

AFTERNOON SNACK:

¼ CUP TOASTED SOY NUTS

DINNER:

FAMILY FUN FONDUE (PAGE 109)

DESSERT:

5 CHOCOLATE-DIPPED STRAWBERRIES (PAGE 137)

DAY 16

BREAKFAST:

PLAIN YOGURT WITH CINNAMON AND BERRIES OR GREEN APPLE SLICES,
    SLIVERED ALMONDS
GREEN TEA

MID-MORNING SNACK:

KALE CHIPS (PAGE 81)

LUNCH:

LEAN TURKEY OR SALMON BURGER
SLICED TOMATO

AFTERNOON SNACK:

PEAR

DINNER:

SPAGHETTI SQUASH SAUTÉ (PAGE 104)

DESSERT:

BAKED APPLE (PAGE 135)

DAY 17

BREAKFAST:

POACHED EGGS WITH TWO SLICES TURKEY BACON

CANTALOUPE OR HONEYDEW WEDGE

GREEN TEA

MID-MORNING SNACK:

½ CUP BLUEBERRIES

LUNCH:

GRILLED SALMON, TROUT, OR HALIBUT

LARGE GREEN SALAD

AFTERNOON SNACK:

GREEN APPLE

DINNER:

LOW-CARB KASHA VARNISHKAS (PAGE 63)

STEAMED BROCCOLI WITH FRESH LEMON JUICE

EVENING SNACK:

TOASTED PUMPKIN SEEDS (PAGE 85)

DAY 18

BREAKFAST:

SUPER SUPPER OMELET (PAGE 112)

GREEN TEA

MID-MORNING SNACK:

SUNFLOWER BUTTER WITH SLICED CUCUMBER

LUNCH:

1 CUP COTTAGE CHEESE

BERRY MEDLEY

SLICED CANTALOUPE

AFTERNOON SNACK:

GUACAMOLE (PAGE 83)

TOMATO SLICES

DINNER:

ROASTED CHICKEN

MOCK POTATOES (PAGE 132)

GREEN SALAD

DESSERT:

GRAPE FREEZE (ABOUT 6 GRAPES; PAGE 134)

DAY 19

BREAKFAST:

SLOW-COOKED OATMEAL WITH ½ CUP BERRIES

MILK

GREEN TEA

MID-MORNING SNACK:

EASY AVOCADO-TURKEY ROLLS (PAGE 84)

LUNCH:

GRILLED SALMON BURGER WITH LIME WEDGE FOR FLAVORING

GRILLED ASPARAGUS WITH OLIVE OIL, FRESHLY GROUND PEPPER, AND
    LEMON JUICE

SLICED TOMATO

AFTERNOON SNACK:

CANTALOUPE WEDGE

DINNER:

LEMONY HUMMUS (PAGE 90)

CUCUMBER-TOMATO SALAD

EVENING SNACK:

PEPPER SALAD (PAGE 82)

DAY 20

BREAKFAST:

BREAKFAST QUINOA (PAGE 64)

MILK, IF DESIRED

CANTALOUPE SLICE

GREEN TEA

MID-MORNING SNACK:

5 ALMOND CRACKERS (PAGE 89)

LUNCH:

LEAN TURKEY BURGER OR QUICK TUNA SALAD (PAGE 101)

TOMATO SLICES

PEPPER SALAD (PAGE 82)

AFTERNOON SNACK:

BIG BERRY BLAST

DINNER:

MINI SPANIS (PAGE 111)

BOK CHOI SALAD WITH 1 TABLESPOON OLIVE OIL AND A SPLASH
    OF VINEGAR

DESSERT:

PEAR CRISP (PAGE 140)

DAY 21

BREAKFAST:

AUTHENTIC PORRIDGE (PAGE 62)

BERRIES

MILK

GREEN TEA

MID-MORNING SNACK:

PEAR

5–10 ALMONDS

LUNCH:

CHOPPED CHICKEN LIVER PÂTÉ (PAGE 118)

PARMA CRISPS (PAGE 88)

AFTERNOON SNACK:

KALE CHIPS (PAGE 81)

DINNER:

BROILED LAMB CHOPS (PAGE 121)

WILTED SPINACH

MOCK POTATOES (PAGE 132)

DESSERT:

MOCK CHOC SHAKE (PAGE 79)

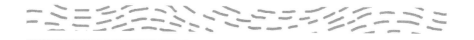

PART TWO

Sugar Detox Recipes

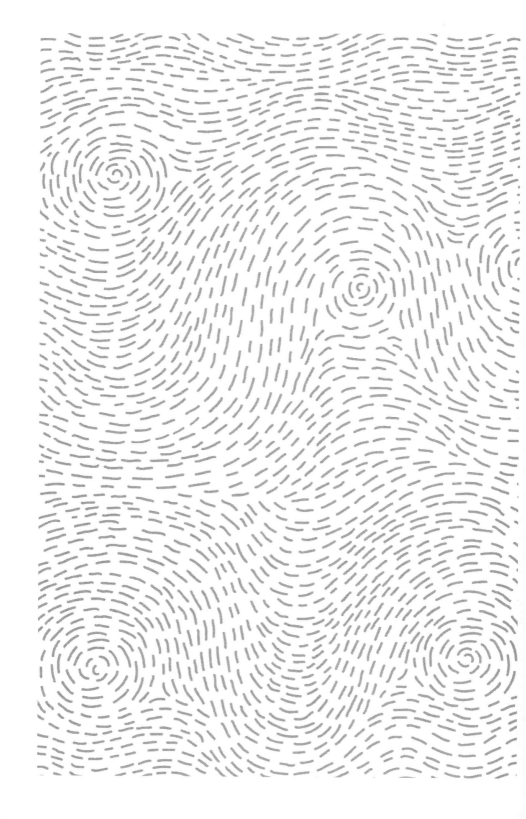

CHAPTER 4

Breakfast

Authentic Porridge

Slow-cooked oatmeal and Irish or Scottish porridge represent two of the permissible grains of sugar-free living. You might find you quite enjoy porridge. It's filling and tasty, and the fact that it takes a few extra minutes to cook might make you feel as if you're really making an effort (but it's not at all hard to make). Here's a from-scratch recipe—you'll probably find the store-bought kind even easier. Consider the milk optional. If you wish, replace the cooking milk with water.

¼ CUP PINHEAD OATMEAL

¼ CUP MEDIUM OATMEAL

½ CUP MILK OR SUGAR-FREE MILK SUBSTITUTE

1 CUP WATER

FRESH BERRIES

ADDITIONAL COLD MILK, FOR SERVING

1. In a large skillet, toast the oats until fragrant. Transfer to a saucepan with milk and water. Bring to a slow boil, stirring frequently. (A wooden spoon is best.)
2. Simmer, stirring, for about 10 to 15 minutes.
3. Cover and let sit for 5 minutes more. Serve with cold milk and berries.

Low-Carb Kasha Varnishkas

SERVES 1

The traditional Russian recipe for kasha varnishkas includes bow-tie pasta. Here's a healthier version you can whip up for breakfast. Kasha is buckwheat groats.

2 TABLESPOONS OIL

1 LARGE ONION, FINELY CHOPPED

1 EGG

1 CUP KASHA

2 CUPS BOILING WATER OR SOUP STOCK

¼ TEASPOON FRESHLY GROUND BLACK PEPPER

1. In a large skillet, heat the oil. Sauté the onions, about 5 minutes. Transfer onion to a paper towel to drain.

2. Meanwhile, in a medium bowl, beat the egg. Stir the kasha into the egg, making sure that all kernels are coated.

3. Pour mixture into heated skillet and cook, stirring, until egg has dried and kernels are separate, about 3 minutes.

4. Boil water or stock and pour over kasha. Add onions and pepper. Cover and simmer until liquid has been absorbed, about 10 to 15 minutes.

Breakfast Quinoa

SERVES 1

For those who miss sugary morning cereals, this is a tasty substitute. Another breakfast recipe that subverts convention. Feel free to experiment with slivered nuts and any kind of berries for even more variety.

QUINOA FLAKES
UNSWEETENED MILK
1 APPLE, SLICED
GROUND CINNAMON

Prepare quinoa flakes according to package directions. Add milk and top with apple slices and cinnamon. Serve warm.

Peach Nut Parfait

SERVES 1

This quick and creamy dessert or snack makes a passable pudding substitute.

1 CUP PLAIN UNSWEETENED YOGURT (REGULAR OR GREEK), DIVIDED

1 PEACH, PITTED AND SLICED, DIVIDED

¼ CUP SLIVERED ALMONDS, DIVIDED

In the bottom of a parfait glass (or comparable dish), place a layer of plain yogurt. Add some sliced peaches and slivered almonds. Add another layer of yogurt, and so on, until finished.

Yogurt Supreme

SERVES 1

Plain yogurt doesn't have to be yucky. Dress it up a bit.

1 CUP PLAIN UNSWEETENED YOGURT (REGULAR OR GREEK)
2 TEASPOONS GROUND CINNAMON
¼ CUP FRESH BLUEBERRIES (OR STRAWBERRIES, IF YOU PREFER)
¼ CUP SLIVERED ALMONDS (OPTIONAL)

1. In a small serving bowl, combine all ingredients.

2. Serve with sliced green apples or melon.

Busy Morning "Brekkie"

It happens to all of us: Some days, we're too busy to prepare a decent meal. When you find yourself rushed at breakfast time, don't skip it and skip out the door. Choose your own portions here, within reason, and fill a thermos with green tea to take with you.

½ CANTALOUPE, SEEDS REMOVED
COTTAGE CHEESE
STRAWBERRIES, SLICED
BLUEBERRIES

Top melon half with cottage cheese and berries.

Breakfast Egg Salad

SERVES 4

Egg salad for breakfast? Well, why not? This recipe lends variety—and deliciousness—to the tried-and-true egg.

4 HARD-BOILED EGGS

1 SCANT TABLESPOON MAYONNAISE

1 TEASPOON DRIED DILL WEED

1 TEASPOON PAPRIKA (OPTIONAL)

¼ RED ONION, MINCED

FRESHLY GROUND BLACK PEPPER, TO TASTE

1. Allow the eggs to cool; then peel and put through large press, or simply chop.

2. In a large bowl, combine eggs with other remaining ingredients.

3. Serve with celery sticks, lettuce leaves, tomato slices, or bell pepper slices, or eat as is.

Easy Breezy Frittata

SERVES 4

A ratatouille-like version of the neoclassic favorite.

4 EGGS
¼ CUP MILK OR TOMATO JUICE
¼ TEASPOON DRIED THYME
FRESHLY GROUND PEPPER, TO TASTE
1 CUP (TOTAL) CHOPPED TOMATOES, BELL PEPPER STRIPS, ZUCCHINI, AND
    BROCCOLI
2 TABLESPOONS VEGETABLE OIL

1. In medium bowl, beat eggs, milk, thyme, and pepper. Add vegetables.
    Mix well.

2. In large skillet, heat the oil. Add mixture and cook on medium-low until
    eggs are set, or nearly so, about 10 minutes. Turn off heat, but leave pan
    on burner so that the eggs continue to cook for a few more minutes.

Baked Egg

When you want something a little different, but not too much ...

1 SLICE LEAN TURKEY BACON

1 TABLESPOON PLAIN YOGURT

1 TOMATO, DICED

1 EGG

¼ CUP FRESH CHOPPED BASIL OR OREGANO

FRESHLY GROUND BLACK PEPPER, TO TASTE (OPTIONAL)

1. Preheat oven to 400°F.

2. Place turkey bacon around inner rim of a ramekin. Place the yogurt in the center of the dish and top with the diced tomato. Crack the egg and pour it into the middle of the dish. Top with basil and pepper, if using.

3. Bake until the egg is fully cooked, at least 15 minutes. (Test the center for doneness before eating.)

Green Eggs and Ham

SERVES 2

Especially fun for kids, this recipe is sure to find favor with the adults in your life, too!

1 CUP SPINACH LEAVES

6 EGGS

2 TABLESPOONS FRESHLY CHOPPED ONION

1 TABLESPOON MILK

FRESHLY GROUND BLACK PEPPER, TO TASTE

OIL, FOR COOKING

2 PIECES LEAN HAM, TO SERVE

1. Wash spinach and remove large stems.

2. In a blender, combine eggs, onion, spinach, milk, and pepper and blend thoroughly. Mixture should be green.

3. In a large skillet, heat oil over medium-low heat. Pour in egg mixture and cook, stirring gently, until eggs are cooked thoroughly. Add more pepper, if desired. Serve with ham slice.

Almond Pancakes

SERVES 2

Substitutions make these pancakes very passable stand-ins for the real thing. Top with a little butter, if you wish—but no syrup!

1 CUP ALMOND FLOUR

¼ TEASPOON BAKING SODA

¼ TEASPOON GROUND CINNAMON (OPTIONAL)

4 EGGS

1 TEASPOON VANILLA EXTRACT

BUTTER (OPTIONAL)

1. In a large bowl, whisk dry ingredients.

2. Add eggs and vanilla, and whisk until well blended.

3. Heat a large skillet or pancake griddle. Drop batter by spoonfuls onto skillet or griddle. When browned, turn and cook completely on other side. Top with a little butter if you wish.

Breakfast Roundies

YIELDS TWO DOZEN

2½ CUP ALMOND FLOUR

½ TEASPOON BAKING SODA

½ CUP UNSALTED BUTTER, MELTED, OR VEGETABLE OIL OR COCONUT OIL

ABOUT 2 CUPS NUTS, SUNFLOWER SEEDS, OR A COMBINATION

1 EGG OR ¼ CUP PLAIN YOGURT

1 TABLESPOON VANILLA EXTRACT

1. In a large bowl, thoroughly combine all ingredients except for egg and vanilla. Then add egg and vanilla to make a dough.

2. Roll the dough into a log and freeze for about an hour.

3. Preheat oven to 350°F.

4. Slice frozen dough into quarter-inch rounds. Place on nonstick cookie sheet and bake 12 to 15 minutes, or until browned around the edges.

Tofu Scramble

Try this variation on classic scrambled eggs.

1 BLOCK TOFU, DRAINED AND PRESSED

2 TABLESPOONS COOKING OIL, BUTTER, OR MARGARINE

½ YELLOW ONION, DICED

½ GREEN BELL PEPPER, DICED

1 TEASPOON GARLIC POWDER

1 TEASPOON ONION POWDER

1 TABLESPOON SOY SAUCE

2 TABLESPOONS NUTRITIONAL YEAST

½ TEASPOON GROUND TURMERIC (OPTIONAL)

1. Crumble the tofu, using a fork.

2. In a large skillet, heat the cooking oil.

3. Sauté the tofu with onion and pepper for about 5 minutes, stirring.

4. Add remaining ingredients, reduce heat, and cook at least 5 more minutes. Make sure tofu is cooked thoroughly.

Breakfast Salmon

Although you might not be accustomed to eating fish for breakfast, it's a great way to get protein, nourishment, and "brain food" first thing. You might find you feel better than you used to, and perform better at work, too. Add a green vegetable, such as quickly steamed broccoli, and a plate of plain quinoa for a complete meal.

¼ CUP SOY SAUCE
1 TABLESPOON TOASTED SESAME OIL
1 TABLESPOON FRESH GINGER, GRATED
2 GARLIC CLOVES, MINCED
2 POUNDS SALMON, CUT INTO ½-POUND PIECES
LEMON WEDGES, TO SERVE

1. In a small bowl, combine all ingredients except for the fish and lemon wedges.

2. Place salmon in a glass baking dish, skin side up (as for baked chicken). Pour marinade over fish, and refrigerate about 2 hours.

3. Preheat the oven to 350°F. Bake until fish is cooked through, 30 to 45 minutes. Serve with lemon wedges.

Turkey Sausage Patties

MAKES ABOUT 8

If you want to try your hand at making your own, you might enjoy these sugar-free patties.

1 POUND LEAN GROUND TURKEY
½ TEASPOON DRIED BASIL LEAF
1 TEASPOON GROUND CORIANDER
½ TEASPOON GROUND CUMIN
½ TEASPOON GARLIC POWDER
½ TEASPOON DRIED OREGANO
1 TEASPOON PAPRIKA
½ TEASPOON CAYENNE PEPPER
DASH OF FRESHLY GROUND BLACK PEPPER
½ CUP CHICKEN BROTH
OIL, FOR COOKING

1. In a large bowl, mix turkey and spices. Add broth and mix well.

2. Form into patties, about ¾ inch thick.

3. Heat a large skillet over medium heat. Cook patties about 7 to 8 minutes. Turn patties and cook on other side until completely cooked.

CHAPTER 5

Snacks

Broiled Grapefruit

This quirky snack rose to its greatest fame in the 1960s. Today, it's one more tool in the dieter's lunchbox!

½ GRAPEFRUIT
GROUND CINNAMON

1. Preheat broiler.

2. Cut around grapefruit sections with a knife to loosen.

3. Sprinkle cinnamon on top.

4. Broil in oven for about 5 minutes. Serve warm.

Mock Choc Shake

When you're ready for a little dairy or sweet fruit—or you're missing chocolate— try this creamy milkshake.

8 OUNCES MILK (WHOLE, 2 PERCENT, OR 1 PERCENT)
½ CUP UNSWEETENED COCOA POWDER
1 SMALL BANANA
PINCH OF GROUND CINNAMON (OPTIONAL)

Blend all ingredients thoroughly for about a minute, or until smooth.

Big Berry Blast

This is a simple, versatile smoothie that packs a big, fruity wallop.

8 OUNCES MILK, ANY KIND (EXCEPT FOR SWEETENED SOY, RICE,
   OR ALMOND)
1 CUP STRAWBERRIES OR BLUEBERRIES, OR ½ CUP OF EACH
4 OUNCES PLAIN UNSWEETENED YOGURT

Blend all ingredients thoroughly, until smooth.

Kale Chips

Even if you don't love kale yet—and you will—these chips are a tasty way to put this superfood to good use.

1 BUNCH KALE
2 TABLESPOONS OLIVE OIL
SEA SALT

1. Preheat oven to 275°F.

2. Wash and dry kale and remove ribs. Cut into snack-size pieces.

3. Arrange kale on baking sheet. Drizzle with olive oil and salt, and turn to coat.

4. Bake until crisp, about 20 minutes, turning once during baking.

Pepper Salad

SERVES 4

If there's a more perfect food than sautéed peppers, we don't want to know about it.

1 RED BELL PEPPER

1 YELLOW BELL PEPPER

1 GREEN BELL PEPPER

1 ORANGE BELL PEPPER (OPTIONAL)

1 LEEK

1 GARLIC CLOVE (OPTIONAL)

FRESHLY GROUND BLACK PEPPER, TO TASTE (OPTIONAL)

OLIVE OIL, FOR SAUTÉING

1. Clean and slice peppers and leek. Slice garlic thinly, or mince.

2. In a large skillet, sauté all ingredients in olive oil, until peppers and leeks are crisp or soft, depending on how you like them. Add ground pepper, if desired.

Guacamole

Basic guacamole is just mashed avocados and a dash of salt. Feel free to create your own healthful variations. You can also make larger quantities to store in the refrigerator. But use your guacamole on the same day you make it—it can quickly become unappetizing. Add a bit of chopped hot pepper if you like it spicy.

1 RIPE AVOCADO

½ SMALL WHITE ONION, SLICED THINLY OR CHOPPED INTO VERY
    SMALL PIECES

1 SMALL TOMATO, DICED

FRESHLY GROUND BLACK PEPPER

LEMON JUICE (OPTIONAL)

1. In a large bowl, mash avocado thoroughly. Add the rest of the ingredients and combine well.

2. Serve with celery sticks. (Or eat it with a fork. No one will think less of you.)

Easy Avocado-Turkey Rolls

YIELDS 1 SERVING FOR EACH TURKEY AND AVOCADO
SLICE USED

One thing virtually all successful diets offer is convenience.

ROASTED TURKEY SLICES
FRESHLY CUT AVOCADO SLICES

Top each turkey slice with an avocado slice. Roll up. Repeat for additional rolls.

Toasted Pumpkin Seeds

YIELDS 6–12 SERVINGS

This childhood staple satisfies the desire for something crunchy. Feel free to experiment with various herbs and spices.

1 PUMPKIN
OLIVE OIL
SALT

1. Cut open pumpkin. Scoop out and thoroughly clean pumpkin seeds by placing them in a colander and running cold tap water over them.

2. Preheat oven to 300°F.

3. Roast seeds on oiled baking sheet for 30 minutes.

4. Remove from oven and toss with olive oil and a little salt. Return to oven. Bake for about 20 minutes, until crisp.

Roasted Nuts

Crunchy, flavorful, and another "secret weapon" in the war against sugar.

1 CUP (8 OUNCES) RAW WALNUTS, ALMONDS, PECANS, CASHEWS,
    OR A COMBINATION
1 TABLESPOON GROUND CINNAMON

1. Preheat oven to 350°F.

2. Place nuts on baking sheet or in oven-safe dish. Sprinkle cinnamon over nuts and shake pan to distribute evenly.

3. Roast for about 10 minutes or to desired level of doneness.

4. Wait until cooled; then transfer to airtight container and refrigerate. Use within a few days or freeze.

Spiced Nuts

Your home will smell heavenly and you'll feel like an accomplished cook!

½ TEASPOON GROUND CINNAMON

1 TEASPOON GROUND GINGER

1½ TEASPOONS VANILLA EXTRACT

1½ TEASPOONS OLIVE OIL

4 OUNCES EACH RAW WALNUTS, PECANS, AND CASHEWS, SHELLED AND BROKEN INTO PIECES

1. Preheat oven to 175°F.

2. In a large bowl, combine cinnamon, ginger, vanilla, and oil. Add nuts and mix to coat. Spoon nuts onto baking sheet and bake for about 10 to 12 minutes. Cool and serve.

3. Store remainder in airtight container. Use within 1 week or freeze.

Parma Crisps

This one-ingredient recipe couldn't be easier—but beware of the fat and salt. Don't eat too many in one sitting.

½ CUP GRATED PARMESAN CHEESE

1. Preheat oven to 400°F.

2. On a baking sheet, pour the cheese 1 tablespoon at a time to form small circles or mounds, spacing about half an inch apart.

3. Bake until golden and crisp, 3 to 5 minutes. Let cool.

Almond Crackers

Almonds have a natural sweetness that really comes out in these crackers.

2 CUPS ALMOND FLOUR
1 EGG
1 TABLESPOON OLIVE OIL

1. Preheat the oven to 350°F.

2. In a large bowl, combine all ingredients. Mix well.

3. Form into a dough and roll out. You might want to do this in two or three batches.

4. Use a knife or pizza wheel to form into crackers.

5. Bake for about 15 minutes, or until crackers begin to brown. Let cool thoroughly; then break crackers apart.

Lemony Hummus

SERVES 2

This delicious Middle Eastern staple is packed with protein and flavor. Whip up a batch for a snack, or serve with salad to make it more of a meal. Goes well with pepper strips or cucumber, or over lettuce.

2¾ CUPS WATER
¼ TEASPOON GROUND CUMIN
¼ TEASPOON FENNEL SEEDS
RED PEPPER FLAKES
5 TABLESPOONS OLIVE OIL, DIVIDED
¾ CUP CHICKPEA FLOUR
¼ CUP TAHINI
1 LEMON
¼ CUP CHOPPED FRESH PARSLEY

1. In a medium saucepan, simmer the water. Meanwhile, in a skillet, toast the cumin and fennel seeds; add red pepper flakes and 2 tablespoons oil. Cook for about 30 seconds. Set aside.

2. Whisk chickpea flour into water and form a paste. Cook for about 2 minutes. Puree paste with tahini and remaining olive oil, and squeeze in as much juice as you can get from the lemon. Top with cumin mixture and parsley, but do not blend. Serve warm or chilled.

CHAPTER 6

Soups and Salads

Basic Gazpacho

A great example of a classic dish that doesn't need sugar or other sweeteners. Perfect on hot summer days.

JUICE OF 1 LEMON

⅓ CUP OLIVE OIL

6 TO 8 TOMATOES (IDEALLY, ROMA OR PLUM), CHOPPED

1 LARGE CUCUMBER, CHOPPED

CHOPPED CILANTRO (IDEALLY FRESH)

2 CLOVES GARLIC

1 LARGE WHITE ONION, ½ CHOPPED FINE AND ½ CHOPPED INTO
   ¼-INCH CHUNKS

FRESHLY GROUND BLACK PEPPER

SALT (OPTIONAL)

1. Pour lemon juice and oil into blender.

2. Add tomatoes, cucumber, cilantro, garlic, onion, and pepper.

3. Blend on a medium setting so that the result is a chunky soup. Add salt, if using.

4. Serve cold. (Parma Crisps make a nice accompaniment, page 88.)

Lentil Soup

SERVES 2

A hearty and heartwarming dish, perfect for detoxers and other dieters.

2 TABLESPOONS OLIVE OIL

1 CLOVE GARLIC, CRUSHED

1 MEDIUM ONION, CHOPPED

1 CUP CARROTS, CHOPPED (OR SUBSTITUTE SPINACH, KALE, CHOPPED
   ZUCCHINI, ETC.), IF DOING GRADUAL DETOX

2 STICKS CELERY, CHOPPED

½ CUP LENTILS, RINSED AND DRAINED

1 TABLESPOON CHOPPED FRESH PARSLEY

1 BAY LEAF

FRESHLY GROUND BLACK PEPPER, TO TASTE (OPTIONAL)

2½ CUPS VEGETABLE STOCK OR WATER, OR 2 CUPS WATER AND ¼ CUP
   SOY SAUCE

1. In large saucepan or stockpot, heat the oil.

2. Add garlic and onion, and sauté until translucent. Add carrots, if using,
   and celery. Cook for about 10 minutes.

3. Add lentils, parsley, bay leaf, and pepper, if using. Stir and add stock.
   Bring almost to boiling. Reduce heat. Cover and simmer for about an
   hour and a half. Remove bay leaf before serving.

Chelsea Chicken Soup

SERVES 4

Chicken soup is infinitely adaptable. Add the kasha or barley if you miss chicken-noodle or chicken rice soup, or if you're feeling underfed. Use any approved vegetable in place of, or in addition to, those listed here.

1 WHOLE CHICKEN, CUT INTO EIGHTHS

3 OR 4 CELERY STALKS, CLEANED AND CHOPPED

¼ CUP SPINACH, KALE, OR CHARD, CHOPPED OR TORN INTO
    BITE-SIZE PIECES

1 LARGE ONION, QUARTERED

3 TO 4 GARLIC CLOVES, MINCED

¼ CUP SOY SAUCE

FRESHLY GROUND BLACK PEPPER, TO TASTE

1 TEASPOON DRIED PARSLEY

DILL WEED, FRESH OR DRIED: A FEW HANDFULS, CHOPPED, IF USING
    FRESH; ABOUT 1 TABLESPOON IF DRIED

½ CUP LENTILS (OPTIONAL)

½ CUP UNCOOKED QUINOA (OPTIONAL)

1. Fill a large stockpot or Dutch oven with water, and add all ingredients except for the dill and quinoa or lentils, if using.

2. Heat to boiling; then reduce heat to simmer.

3. Cover and cook for 1 hour; then add dill and rinsed quinoa or lentils (or both), if using.

4. Simmer an additional 30–60 minutes; then check chicken for doneness.

Pear & Pom Salad

SERVES 2

An attractive salad, ideal for company, but easy enough to make just for you.

3 CUPS ROMAINE LETTUCE, CLEANED AND TORN INTO BITE-SIZE PIECES
1 BARTLETT OR ANJOU PEAR
⅓ CUP POMEGRANATE SEEDS
1 TABLESPOON VEGETABLE OIL
2 TABLESPOONS POMEGRANATE JUICE
1 TABLESPOON LEMON JUICE
1 TEASPOON SUGAR-FREE MUSTARD
FRESHLY GROUND BLACK PEPPER, TO TASTE

1. Divide lettuce between two bowls.

2. Slice pears. Distribute pear slices and pomegranate seeds among bowls and mix gently.

3. In small saucepan over high heat, cook vegetable oil, pomegranate juice, lemon juice, mustard, and pepper. Bring to a boil; reduce heat and simmer, stirring frequently, about 2 minutes. (Mixture should thicken.)

4. Pour dressing over the salads. Serve immediately.

Super Supper Salad

SERVES 2

The beauty of the supper salad is that you can add or subtract from it as you see fit. Experiment with different types of lettuce and other green vegetables, olives, avocados, and so on. You can even add lean cooked chicken, turkey, or ham.

1 HEAD ROMAINE LETTUCE, WASHED AND TORN INTO BITE-SIZE PIECES

½ CUP SPINACH, WASHED

½ CUP ARUGULA, WASHED

1 RADISH, SLICED

1 CUCUMBER, SLICED

1 RED BELL PEPPER, SLICED

1 HEAD CHOPPED BROCCOLI

2 AVOCADOS, SLICED

¼ CUP CHOPPED PARSLEY (CURLY OR FLAT)

SPRINKLE OF FETA CHEESE (OPTIONAL), IF YOU'RE ON THE GRADUAL DETOX

1 PINCH FRESHLY GROUND BLACK PEPPER

2 HARD-COOKED EGGS, SLICED

1 TABLESPOON OLIVE OIL

½ TEASPOON LEMON JUICE

1. In a large bowl, combine all ingredients except for eggs, oil, and lemon juice. Toss lightly.

2. Top with egg slices, oil, and lemon juice.

Salad Sauté

SERVES 1

Who says lettuce has to be eaten cold? This recipe, too, can be altered to suit your tastes. Feel free to experiment with different vegetable combinations.

OLIVE OIL, FOR SAUTÉING

1 GARLIC CLOVE, MINCED (OPTIONAL)

½ CUP BROCCOLI FLORETS

½ CUP CAULIFLOWER FLORETS

1 CUP ROMAINE LETTUCE, TORN INTO BITE-SIZE PIECES

¼ CUP CHOPPED FRESH PARSLEY

1 LARGE TOMATO, CHOPPED

THINLY SLICED RED AND GREEN BELL PEPPER STRIPS

½ CUP SLICED MUSHROOMS

BULB OF 1 SCALLION, WASHED AND MINCED

FRESHLY GROUND BLACK PEPPER, TO TASTE (OPTIONAL)

1. In a large skillet, warm the oil. Add garlic, if using, and then florets and remaining vegetables.

2. Sauté until garlic, peppers, and florets are cooked, and lettuce is wilted. Add pepper, if using.

Cold Quinoa Salad

SERVES 2

An exotic but not terribly difficult dish using versatile and satisfying quinoa.

1 CUP QUINOA

4 RADISHES

½ MEDIUM-SIZE FENNEL BULB, CORED

ZEST OF 2 LEMONS, GRATED FINELY

JUICE FROM 1 LEMON

2 TABLESPOONS OLIVE OR VEGETABLE OIL

FRESHLY GROUND BLACK PEPPER, TO TASTE (OPTIONAL)

1. Thoroughly rinse quinoa and prepare according to package directions. Meanwhile, slice radishes and fennel bulb thinly and refrigerate until crisp.

2. Combine lemon zest and juice with oil. Add quinoa and toss. Top with radish and fennel slices. Add pepper, if using.

Red Lentil Salad

Red lentils cook fastest of all the lentils. Prepare this nourishing dish when you're very hungry or pressed for time.

1 CUP RED LENTILS

⅓ CUP BALSAMIC VINEGAR

2 TABLESPOONS OLIVE OIL

2 CLOVES GARLIC, MINCED

¾ CUP CHOPPED YELLOW BELL PEPPERS

¾ CUP SLICED SCALLIONS

¾ CUP CHERRY TOMATOES, CUT INTO HALVES

1 CUCUMBER, CHOPPED

½ CUP CHOPPED FRESH BASIL

FRESHLY GROUND BLACK PEPPER, TO TASTE (OPTIONAL)

1. Rinse and drain lentils. Cook according to package directions, until just soft.

2. In a small bowl, combine vinegar, oil, and garlic. Pour over lentils. Toss to coat and let stand. Add remaining ingredients. Season with pepper, if desired. Stir to combine.

Tofu Salad

SERVES 2

Once again, tofu demonstrates its remarkable versatility.

3 TABLESPOONS CANOLA OIL

2 TABLESPOONS RICE WINE VINEGAR

2 TEASPOONS SOY SAUCE

1 TEASPOON SESAME OIL

1 TEASPOON FRESH GINGER, MINCED

1 (14-OUNCE) PACKAGE EXTRA-FIRM TOFU, RINSED, PATTED DRY,
    AND CUT INTO 1-INCH CUBES

8 CUPS SALAD GREENS

1 LARGE CUCUMBER, CHOPPED

¼ OF A SAVOY CABBAGE, SLICED THINLY

1. In a large bowl, whisk together canola oil, vinegar, soy sauce, sesame oil, and ginger.

2. Place 2 tablespoons of the mixture in skillet and add tofu. Cook on medium-high heat, turning every 2 to 3 minutes, until golden brown (about 15 minutes).

4. Remove from heat; add 1 tablespoon of the mixture to the skillet. Stir to coat.

5. Toss remaining ingredients with remaining dressing and place tofu on top. Serve immediately.

Quick Tuna Salad

The suburban mom's classic.

1 CAN OR POUCH OF TUNA, OR A FRESHLY COOKED PIECE OF TUNA
  STEAK, ABOUT 6 OUNCES
1 CELERY RIB, WASHED AND DICED THINLY
1 SCALLION BULB, WASHED AND SLICED THINLY
½ CUP SUGAR-FREE MAYONNAISE OR SALAD DRESSING
1 TEASPOON LEMON JUICE (OPTIONAL)
DASH BLACK OR CAYENNE PEPPER
LETTUCE, ANY KIND

1. In a large bowl, thoroughly combine all ingredients except lettuce.

2. Serve over lettuce.

CHAPTER 7

Main Courses

Mock Pasta Ribbons

YIELD DEPENDS ON QUANTITIES USED

Craving carbs? Relax. These delicious ribbons look and "act" almost like the real thing. Use summer squash for added believability!

USE ANY QUANTITY OF THE FOLLOWING AS YOU WISH:

SUMMER SQUASH, ZUCCHINI, OR BOTH

OLIVE OIL, FOR SAUTÉING

RED TOMATOES, CHOPPED INTO BITE-SIZE PIECES

SPINACH OR ARUGULA

BROCCOLI, CHOPPED INTO BITE-SIZE PIECES

GARLIC, FINELY MINCED

FRESHLY GROUND BLACK PEPPER, TO TASTE

1. Preheat the oven to 200°F.

2. Drive a skewer through one end of squash, all the way down and out the bottom. (The vegetable should look roughly like a violin.) Carefully run a vegetable peeler down the length of the squash for a long, pretty "ribbon." Repeat until all of the squash, except for the very middle, is peeled.

3. Place ribbons on a baking sheet and bake for 5 minutes.

4. In large skillet, heat oil on low. Add all other ingredients. Sauté over medium heat until garlic is translucent and all vegetables are cooked through. Serve immediately with green salad or plain quinoa.

Spaghetti Squash Sauté

Here's another very serviceable carb substitute.

1 MEDIUM TO LARGE SPAGHETTI SQUASH
OLIVE OIL, FOR SAUTÉING
4 TOMATOES, CHOPPED
3 OR 4 GARLIC CLOVES, MINCED
½ CUP FRESH SPINACH OR CHARD, WASHED AND TORN INTO
    BITE-SIZE PIECES
2 HEADS BROCCOLI, CLEANED AND CHOPPED
FRESHLY GROUND BLACK PEPPER, TO TASTE (OPTIONAL)

1. Preheat oven to 375°F.

2. Carefully pierce the cleaned outside of the whole squash with the tines of a fork or sharp knife. Bake for about an hour.

3. Remove from oven carefully and, using a sharp knife, cut lengthwise. Remove seeds. Let cool. Using a fork, scrape the spaghetti-like flesh from the squash.

4. In large frying pan or skillet, warm the oil. Add squash and sauté. Add tomatoes, garlic, spinach, broccoli, and pepper, if using. Sauté until squash is soft and translucent and garlic and vegetables are cooked. Serve with green salad.

Mock Breaded Eggplant

SERVES 4-6

This is a fun recipe to make with kids, as quantities don't need to be exact. You can substitute green tomatoes for the eggplant; farmers' markets and farm stands are great places to find them, from late August to late October. You can also use sliced zucchini instead of eggplant for an unusual side dish. (If you like, you can substitute ¼ cup of unflavored, unsweetened yogurt or a little water or milk for the egg. If using tomatoes, you can skip this step altogether, as the tomato's natural stickiness will hold the coating unassisted.)

FALAFEL MIX (SUCH AS FANTASTIC FOODS BRAND)
1 MEDIUM EGGPLANT OR 5 LARGE GREEN TOMATOES, THINLY SLICED
1 EGG OR EGG WHITE, MIXED WITH A LITTLE WATER
OLIVE OIL, FOR FRYING
FINELY CHOPPED PARSLEY FOR GARNISH (OPTIONAL)

1. Shake about a ½ cup (to start) of the falafel mix onto a plate. Dip the eggplant slices into the egg or yogurt to coat, then into the falafel mix.

2. Fry in oil until well cooked on both sides. Drain on paper towels.

3. Garnish with parsley and serve with plain quinoa or Mock Pasta Ribbons (page 103) and steamed broccoli with lemon juice.

Ratatouille

Ratatouille is a longtime vegetarian staple, but carnivores and omnivores will probably find they like it, too.

¼ CUP OLIVE OIL, PLUS MORE AS NEEDED

1½ CUPS DICED ONIONS

1 TEASPOON GARLIC, MINCED

2 CUPS CUBED EGGPLANT

½ TEASPOON FRESH THYME LEAVES

1 CUP DICED GREEN BELL PEPPERS

1 CUP DICED RED BELL PEPPERS

1 CUP DICED ZUCCHINI

1 CUP DICED SUMMER SQUASH

1½ CUPS CHOPPED TOMATOES

1 TABLESPOON FINELY CUT FRESH BASIL LEAVES

1 TABLESPOON CHOPPED FRESH PARSLEY LEAVES

FRESHLY GROUND BLACK PEPPER

1. In a large skillet, heat the oil over medium heat.

2. Add onions and garlic. Cook, stirring, until both are translucent and fragrant, about 5 to 7 minutes.

3. Add eggplant and thyme. Cook, stirring, for about 5 minutes.

4. Add peppers, zucchini, and squash. Cook for 5 minutes.

5. Add remaining ingredients and cook 5 minutes more. Stir and serve.

Soba Stir-Fry

SERVES 1-2

Feel free to substitute the detox-diet-permissible veggies of your choice. Peanut butter increases the protein content, but feel free to omit it, or to substitute another nut butter or even tofu cubes. Make sure to cook soy products thoroughly. (Pure buckwheat noodles contain no flour, but these can be pricey and texturally less desirable than their 70–30 counterparts.)

8 OUNCES SOBA NOODLES
OIL, FOR FRYING
1 TABLESPOON PEANUT BUTTER
1 RED PEPPER, SLICED
½ CUP FRESH SPINACH LEAVES, WASHED
1 CUP CHOPPED BROCCOLI
1 CUP SAVOY CHOPPED CABBAGE
1 GARLIC CLOVE, MINCED (OPTIONAL)
½ TEASPOON FRESH GINGER, GRATED (OPTIONAL)
FRESHLY GROUND BLACK PEPPER (OPTIONAL)

1. Boil noodles according to package directions.

2. In a large skillet, heat the oil. Add the noodles and the rest of the ingredients. Cook, stirring, over medium-low heat, until desired doneness is reached.

Quinoa Vegetable Sauté

SERVES 4

As a grain substitute (actually a kind of seed, although you'd never know it), quinoa can provide the satisfying qualities of rice or other grains.

1 CUP QUINOA

1 TO 2 TABLESPOONS OLIVE OIL, FOR SAUTÉING

1 SLICED YELLOW BELL PEPPER

1 SMALL CHOPPED ONION

1 CLOVE GARLIC (OR MORE, IF DESIRED), MINCED

1 MEDIUM CHOPPED TOMATO

1 HEAD CHOPPED BROCCOLI OR ½ CUP CHOPPED CAULIFLOWER
    (OPTIONAL)

SPRIG OF FRESH PARSLEY OR CILANTRO, CHOPPED

FRESHLY GROUND BLACK PEPPER

1. Prepare quinoa according to package directions.

2. In a large skillet, heat olive oil.

3. Add pepper slices, onion, and garlic. Sauté until onion is translucent and pepper is soft.

4. Add other ingredients and continue to cook until quinoa reaches your preferred level of doneness.

Family Fun Fondue

SERVES 4

Here's a great way to add some fun to a sugar-free diet, especially—but not exclusively—for kids. Most cheese fondue recipes call for Swiss or Gruyère varieties, but those require white wine for liquidity. Alcohol contains sugars— in fact, one older theory holds that alcoholism is caused by sugar addiction!— so you won't find wine here. This cheddar recipe uses milk instead, so it's permissible for gradual detoxers.

2 CUPS CREAM

1 TABLESPOON WORCESTERSHIRE SAUCE

2 TEASPOONS DRY MUSTARD

1½ POUNDS SHREDDED CHEDDAR, MILD OR SHARP

3 TABLESPOONS FLOUR OR A FLOUR SUBSTITUTE

FRESHLY GROUND BLACK PEPPER, TO TASTE

CHERRY TOMATOES

RAW BROCCOLI FLORETS

RAW CAULIFLOWER FLORETS

RAW BUTTON MUSHROOMS

ZUCCHINI SLICES

1. In a large pot, heat cream and Worcestershire sauce over low heat. Add mustard.

2. In a large bowl, mix cheese and flour together. Add to the pot little by little, letting the cheese melt before you add more. Stir. When cheese is melted and bubbling slightly, add pepper, if using. Pour into a fondue pot, if using one, or other comparable serving bowl or pot.

3. Skewer vegetables and dip into fondue.

Crustless Quiche

Another great example of how, with a little modification, you can still enjoy many of the same foods as always.

OIL, FOR SAUTÉING

8 OUNCES FRESH MUSHROOMS, RINSED AND SLICED THINLY

½ TEASPOON GARLIC, MINCED

FRESHLY GROUND BLACK PEPPER, TO TASTE (OPTIONAL)

1 (10-OUNCE) PACKAGE FROZEN SPINACH, THAWED AND DRAINED

2 OUNCES FETA CHEESE, CRUMBLED

4 LARGE EGGS

1 CUP MILK

¼ CUP PARMESAN, GRATED

½ CUP MOZZARELLA, SHREDDED

1. Preheat oven to 350°F.

2. In a large skillet, heat the oil. Add mushrooms, garlic, and pepper, if using. Sauté over medium-high heat for about 5 to 7 minutes.

3. Grease a pie plate with unsalted butter and spread the spinach over the bottom. Add mushroom mixture and feta.

4. In a medium bowl, whisk together eggs until smooth. Add milk, Parmesan, and pepper, if using. Pour mixture into dish and sprinkle with mozzarella.

5. Bake for 45 minutes and test for doneness: the quiche should be golden brown and a knife inserted into the center should come out clean. If not yet done, return dish to oven and bake for up to 15 minutes. Slice and serve.

Mini Spanis

SERVES 6 OR MORE

This spanakopita recipe uses tapioca flour, so it's grain-free, too.

2 TABLESPOONS PINE NUTS

2 (7.5-OUNCE) BOXES CHEBE FOCACCIA MIX

6 TABLESPOONS OLIVE OIL, DIVIDED

4 LARGE EGGS

½ CUP WATER

1 CUP PARMESAN CHEESE, GRATED

1 SMALL WHITE ONION, CHOPPED

2 SCALLIONS, CLEANED AND MINCED

1 (10-OUNCE) BOX FROZEN SPINACH, THAWED

4 OUNCES CRUMBLED FETA CHEESE

½ CUP RICOTTA CHEESE

½ TEASPOON FRESHLY GROUND BLACK PEPPER

½ TEASPOON FRESHLY GRATED NUTMEG

1. Preheat oven to 375°F.

2. Grease 24 muffin cups with unsalted butter, or use nonstick cups or cooking spray.

3. In a large skillet over medium heat, toast pine nuts, stirring, about 3 or 4 minutes, until lightly browned. Remove from skillet.

4. Combine focaccia mix, 4 tablespoons oil, eggs, water, and Parmesan in large bowl. Knead until smooth (1 or 2 minutes). Divide dough into balls. Place each ball into a muffin cup. Make an indentation in each.

5. In a large skillet, heat 2 remaining tablespoons oil on medium-high. Add onion and cook, stirring, until translucent (about 5 minutes). Add scallions and cook for an additional minute. Drain spinach and add it to the skillet. Cook, stirring, until the spinach is dry.

6. In a large bowl, combine the spinach mixture with pine nuts, feta, ricotta, pepper, and nutmeg. Spoon into indented dough cups and bake for 15 minutes or until lightly browned and dry in center.

Super Supper Omelet

If omelet making is difficult for you, you can make this scrambled-eggs-and-veggies dish and no one will be the wiser. A word about oil: olive oil, though expensive, will impart a lovely smoothness to your skin. (On the other hand, it's not low in calories, so be careful not to overuse it if you're watching your weight.) It may be substituted for canola oil in this and other recipes. Take care with any cooking oil not to overheat it, or it can spatter and smoke. This recipe makes one omelet.

When you have fish for breakfast, why not enjoy a veggie-filled omelet later on?

CANOLA OIL, FOR FRYING

3 EGGS

RED BELL PEPPER, SLICED

A FEW SPRIGS PARSLEY

¼ CUP CHOPPED BROCCOLI

FRESHLY GROUND BLACK PEPPER, TO TASTE

1. In a medium skillet, warm the oil. Separate two of the eggs. In a bowl, thoroughly mix one whole egg with two whites. Discard extra yolks.

2. Pour mixture into skillet. With a spatula, poke the edges of the omelet toward the center. Then tilt the pan so that the less-cooked parts of the omelet flow back toward the outer edges. Repeat until the omelet sets. Use the spatula to flip it over so that it cooks on the other side. Meanwhile, add the remaining ingredients and fold the omelet over once gently.

3. Turn off the heat and let the omelet finish cooking until heated through.

4. Flip onto a plate and serve with plain quinoa and steamed green vegetable of your choice.

Homemade Falafel

Turn up the spice quantity if you like it hot; reduce the spices if you don't.

1 CUP CHICKPEA FLOUR

¼ TEASPOON BAKING SODA

¼ TEASPOON GROUND CUMIN

¼ TEASPOON GROUND CORIANDER

¼ TEASPOON YELLOW CURRY POWDER

½ TEASPOON GARLIC POWDER

¼ TEASPOON ONION POWDER

2 TEASPOONS LEMON JUICE

½ CUP HOT WATER

ABOUT ¼ CUP OLIVE OIL, FOR FRYING

1. Thoroughly mix the dry ingredients. Then add lemon juice and hot water, and mix well. Let stand 10 minutes.

2. In a large skillet, heat enough olive oil to cover the bottom. Carefully drop batter into oil by spoonfuls. Cook for about 2 minutes; then flip patties and cook for 2 minutes more. Drain and serve over lettuce and tomato slices.

Szechuan Tofu

SERVES 4

A good protein source for vegetarians and omnivores alike. Dial down the spices if you prefer a milder flavor.

½ CUP WATER, DIVIDED

¼ CUP SOY SAUCE

1 TABLESPOON TOMATO PASTE

2 TEASPOONS BALSAMIC VINEGAR

¼ TO ½ TEASPOON CRUSHED RED PEPPER FLAKES

2 TABLESPOONS PLUS 1 TEASPOON CORNSTARCH

1 (14-OUNCE) PACKAGE EXTRA-FIRM TOFU, DRAINED AND CUBED

2 TABLESPOONS CANOLA OIL, DIVIDED

4 CUPS GREEN BEANS, RINSED, TRIMMED, AND HALVED

4 CLOVES GARLIC, MINCED

2 TEASPOONS FRESH GINGER, GRATED

1. In a bowl, whisk together half of the water with the soy sauce, tomato paste, vinegar, pepper flakes, and 1 teaspoon cornstarch. Dust the tofu with remaining cornstarch to coat.

2. In a wok or large skillet, heat 1 tablespoon oil over medium heat. Add tofu and cook for about 2 minutes. Stir gently and continue to cook for 2 to 3 minutes more (tofu should be brown and crisp). Place tofu on a plate, but leave the pan on the stove.

3. Reduce heat to medium. Add the remaining oil, green beans, garlic, and ginger; cook, stirring constantly, for about a minute. Add the remaining water. Cover and cook about 4 minutes more. Stir in reserved soy sauce mixture. Cook, stirring, until thickened (about a minute). Add tofu and heat through, making sure it's cooked thoroughly.

Fish Kebabs

You will need about ten 8- or 10-inch skewers, ideally. Soak wooden skewers in water for 30 minutes before grilling to prevent burning. Great fun on a warm summer night; when outdoor temps drop, just bake it in the oven.

ABOUT 6 OUNCES EACH: SKINLESS SALMON, HALIBUT, AND TUNA STEAKS,
    CUT INTO ½-INCH CUBES (ABOUT 30 PIECES TOTAL)
ZUCCHINI
ONION
MUSHROOMS
TOMATOES
½ CUP OLIVE OIL
1 LARGE LEMON
7 GARLIC CLOVES, MINCED
1 STICK UNSALTED BUTTER, SOFTENED
3 TABLESPOONS CHOPPED THYME LEAVES
1 CUP PLUS 2 TABLESPOONS CHOPPED PARSLEY
FRESHLY GROUND BLACK PEPPER

1. Place fish in large baking dish in refrigerator. Cut vegetables into chunks and set aside, ideally in refrigerator.

2. In a medium bowl, whisk together the rest of the ingredients, except the pepper and parsley. Pour the oil mixture over the fish, sprinkle with pepper and parsley, and refrigerate for at least 30 minutes. Place fish cubes on skewers, alternating them with vegetables.

3. Preheat the grill. Grill kebabs about 3 or 4 minutes on each side, until thoroughly cooked.

Salmon Teriyaki

SERVES 4

Feel free to substitute other kinds of fish or chicken. Just make sure to adjust cooking times accordingly.

¼ CUP SOY SAUCE
1 TABLESPOON SESAME OIL
1 TABLESPOON GINGER, IDEALLY FRESHLY GRATED
2 CLOVES GARLIC, MINCED
2 POUNDS SALMON STEAKS
LEMON WEDGES

1. In a medium bowl, combine all ingredients, except for the fish and lemon. Mix well.

2. Place salmon in a baking dish and cover with the marinade. Refrigerate for at least 2 hours.

3. Preheat oven to 350°F. Bake until thoroughly cooked, but do not overcook.

4. Serve with lemon wedges.

Simple Sea Bass

SERVES 2-3

Few fish are yummier (or, alas, more expensive) than sea bass, and its oils will help keep facial skin dewy. A great dish for slightly special occasions.

PINCH OF GARLIC POWDER

PINCH OF ONION POWDER

PINCH OF PAPRIKA

PINCH OF FRESHLY GROUND BLACK PEPPER

DASH OF LEMON JUICE

2 TABLESPOONS BUTTER (OPTIONAL)

1¼ POUNDS SEA BASS

2 TEASPOONS CHOPPED FRESH PARSLEY (OR SUBSTITUTE ABOUT
   1 TEASPOON DRIED)

1. Preheat oven to 450°F.

2. Combine garlic powder, onion powder, paprika, pepper, lemon juice, and butter, if using, and spread over fish.

3. Bake for about 20 minutes, or until fish flakes easily with a fork. Garnish with parsley and serve.

Chopped Chicken Liver Pâté

Whether you know it as "chopped liver" or by its fancier French name, pâté, you'll find this dish full of protein and flavor—but not cholesterol, as the following recipe omits much of its famous fat.

1 POUND CHICKEN LIVERS
1 CUP FINELY CHOPPED ONION
1 EGG, HARD-BOILED
FRESHLY GROUND BLACK PEPPER

1. In a large pot, simmer enough water for poaching livers.

2. Rinse livers and remove any stringy tendons. Drop into pot and poach until just done. Drain and let cool. Chop thoroughly.

3. Place chopped liver in a large bowl. Add remaining ingredients and mix well.

Lemon-Lime Chicken

SERVES 4

The unexpected lemon and lime flavors elevate this humble oven-roasted chicken to something special enough to serve to company.

JUICE OF 4 LIMES, OR 2 LEMONS AND 2 LIMES

1 CUP CANOLA OIL

3 OR 4 GARLIC CLOVES, OR AS DESIRED, MINCED

¼ CUP FRESH CHOPPED CILANTRO (SUBSTITUTE PARSLEY OR OTHER
    HERB, IF YOU PREFER)

FRESHLY GROUND BLACK PEPPER, TO TASTE

1 WHOLE CHICKEN, CUT INTO EIGHTHS

1. Combine all ingredients except chicken. Place chicken pieces in a roasting pan and pour mixture over it, coating all pieces evenly. Marinate for 2 to 4 hours in the refrigerator.

2. Preheat the oven to 375°F.

3. Bake for about an hour, or until chicken is thoroughly cooked, when juices run clear.

Simple Roasted Chicken

SERVES 4

This chicken recipe makes enough for a family—or you can simply snack on the leftovers the following day.

ONE (3-POUND) WHOLE CHICKEN, GIBLETS REMOVED
FRESHLY GROUND BLACK PEPPER
1 TABLESPOON ONION POWDER
3 OR 4 WHOLE GARLIC CLOVES, PEELED

1. Preheat oven to 350°F.

2. Place chicken in a roasting pan, and sprinkle with pepper and onion powder. Place garlic atop or beside.

3. Bake about an hour and a quarter, occasionally basting with drippings. (Skip this step if you are carefully watching your fat intake.) Chicken should reach a minimum internal temperature of 180°F. Remove from oven when fully cooked.

Broiled Lamb Chops

In the classic style, lamb chops are done when they're a dusty pink inside. Experiment with different spices for variations on this easy and elegant dish.

4 LAMB CHOPS, ABOUT AN INCH THICK
3 TABLESPOONS OLIVE OIL, DIVIDED
1 GARLIC CLOVE, MINCED
2 TEASPOONS ROSEMARY, IDEALLY FRESH
FRESHLY GROUND BLACK PEPPER, TO TASTE

1. Preheat broiler. Place lamb chops in ovenproof dish. Combine half the oil with garlic, rosemary, and pepper, and pour the mixture over lamb chops, turning to coat.

2. Broil for 5 minutes. Turn them over and baste with remaining oil. Cook for another 5 minutes. Test for doneness.

CHAPTER 8

Side Dishes

Oven-Fried Green Beans

YIELD DEPENDS ON QUANTITY USED

Another simple classic for busy or intimidated cooks. Use whatever quantity of fresh string beans you desire.

STRING BEANS

OLIVE OIL FOR DRIZZLING

SALT (OPTIONAL)

1. Preheat the oven to 400°F.

2. Arrange beans in single layer on baking sheet and drizzle liberally with oil. Bake for 10 minutes. Sprinkle with salt, if desired.

Grilled Asparagus

SERVES 4

Elegant, nutritious, and tasty, this simple side has it all.

1 POUND FRESH ASPARAGUS SPEARS, TRIMMED

1 TABLESPOON OLIVE OIL

FRESHLY GROUND BLACK PEPPER, TO TASTE

1. Preheat the grill on high setting.

2. Coat asparagus with oil and pepper. Grill about 2 to 3 minutes, or until done.

Cherry Tomato Sauté

A great recipe for those who are new to the kitchen or whose time is limited.

2 TABLESPOONS OLIVE OIL FOR SAUTÉING
1 PINT CHERRY TOMATOES
1 CLOVE GARLIC OR MORE, MINCED

1. In a large skillet, warm the oil.

2. Add tomatoes and garlic. Turn up the heat and sauté until tomatoes are soft and have begun to burst, and garlic is cooked, 1 or 2 minutes.

Sesame Zucchini

SERVES 1

The sesame seeds in this recipe bring out the zucchini's rich flavor.

1 ZUCCHINI
OLIVE OIL FOR DRIZZLING
SESAME SEEDS

1. Preheat the oven to 400°F.

2. Slice zucchini lengthwise or crosswise. Arrange on baking sheet.

3. Drizzle liberally with oil. Sprinkle with sesame seeds.

4. Bake for about 10 minutes. Carefully remove from oven.

Zucchini and Onions

SERVES 1 PER ZUCCHINI

A definite crowd pleaser, with the added benefit of being quick and easy to prepare. A simple and surprisingly tasty side.

1 ZUCCHINI PER PERSON
1 MEDIUM ONION
1 GARLIC CLOVE
OIL FOR SAUTÉING

1. Slice zucchini, onion, and garlic.

2. Sauté in skillet until onion is translucent, garlic is fragrant, and zucchini is tender.

Roasted Brussels

SERVES 4

Even those who aren't crazy over veggies will probably enjoy these yummy treats. Cooking for a little longer produces a more tender sprout.

1 CUP BRUSSELS SPROUTS
OLIVE OIL
1 GARLIC CLOVE, MINCED

1. Preheat the oven to 350°F.

2. Wash and trim Brussels sprouts and arrange on baking sheet. Drizzle liberally with oil and garlic. Bake until soft, about 35 to 40 minutes.

Down-Home Coleslaw

Most coleslaw recipes use sugar. See if you miss it in this tangy version, which makes enough for a picnic or informal party.

4 CUPS GREEN CABBAGE

4 CUPS RED CABBAGE

1½ TEASPOONS CELERY SEED

9 TEASPOONS UNSWEETENED MUSTARD

3 TABLESPOONS APPLE CIDER VINEGAR

1 CUP MAYONNAISE

FRESHLY GROUND BLACK OR WHITE PEPPER (OPTIONAL)

1. Finely chop cabbage.

2. In a large bowl, whisk together remaining ingredients.

3. Add cabbage and toss to combine. Add pepper, if using.

Broccoli Almondine

SERVES 4

Naturally nutritious and sugar-free, Broccoli Almondine will appeal to the vegetable-phobic and discriminating diners alike.

1½ POUNDS BROCCOLI

½ STICK UNSALTED BUTTER OR 4 TABLESPOONS VEGETABLE OIL

⅓ CUP SLICED ALMONDS

1 TABLESPOON FRESH LEMON JUICE

1. Trim broccoli stems. Cut broccoli into spears. Steam, ideally in a steamer, until tender, but not overcooked, about 10 minutes. Drain and let cool.

2. While the broccoli is steaming, heat the butter in a medium skillet. Sauté the almonds until golden and fragrant, 2 or 3 minutes. Stir in lemon juice. Pour over broccoli.

Cauliflower Tabbouleh

SERVES 4

Sugar-free living need not be boring. This dish has a Middle Eastern flavor. Feel free to experiment with different spices for different tastes.

1 HEAD CAULIFLOWER

2 TOMATOES, DICED

⅓ CUP LEMON JUICE

3 TABLESPOONS OLIVE OIL

2 TABLESPOONS SOY SAUCE

2 SCALLION BULBS, CHOPPED

FRESH PARSLEY, CHOPPED

FRESH MINT, CHOPPED

FRESHLY GROUND BLACK PEPPER (OPTIONAL)

1. Using box grater or food processor, grate cauliflower into small pieces, about the size of rice grains or slightly larger.

2. Place in large bowl. Toss with remaining ingredients.

Mock Potatoes

Cauliflower has a clean, creamy taste that will make you wonder why you bothered eating potatoes in the first place.

1 LARGE HEAD CAULIFLOWER
1 GARLIC CLOVE, MINCED
2 TABLESPOONS OLIVE OIL
1 TO 2 CUPS WATER OR MILK
FRESHLY GROUND BLACK PEPPER OR CAYENNE PEPPER (OPTIONAL)

1. Preheat the oven to 400°F.

2. Cut cauliflower into bite-size pieces and place in large bowl. Add garlic and oil and stir to coat.

3. Place cauliflower in baking pan. Bake until brown around the edges, about 20 minutes. Allow to cool.

4. Place cauliflower in blender or food processor. Blend or pulse with water until mixture resembles mashed potatoes. Serve with pepper, if desired.

CHAPTER 9

Desserts

Grape Freeze

If you believe that the simplest things are the best ... you're in luck!

2 CUPS SEEDLESS RED OR GREEN GRAPES

Freeze grapes for a minimum of 45 minutes. Let stand for 2 minutes at room temperature before serving.

Baked Apple

SERVES 1

1 GRANNY SMITH APPLE (OR AS MANY AS YOU WANT), WASHED AND
SLICED THINLY
1 TABLESPOON GROUND CINNAMON (OR MORE)
¼ TEASPOON GROUND NUTMEG (OPTIONAL)
¼ CUP SLIVERED ALMONDS (OPTIONAL)
BUTTER, FOR DOTTING ON TOP

1. Preheat the oven to 350°F.

2. Arrange apple slices in a pie dish. Top with spices and nuts, if using. Dot butter on top. Bake until cooked through, about 30 minutes.

3. Serve with plain yogurt, if desired.

Frozen Fruit

YIELDS 6–12 SERVINGS

CANTALOUPE SLICE, CUT AWAY FROM THE RIND
HONEYDEW SLICE, CUT AWAY FROM THE RIND
HALF A BANANA, CUT INTO SLICES (IF DOING GRADUAL DETOX)
GROUND CINNAMON

1. Cut melon into bite-size pieces.

2. Cut banana into slices and sprinkle cinnamon on top.

3. Arrange all fruit in a dish. Cover and freeze overnight.

Chocolate-Dipped Strawberries

Like the Mock Choc Shake, this dessert uses the natural sweetness of the fruit to provide the sugar.

3½ OUNCES UNSWEETENED BAKING CHOCOLATE, CHOPPED
1 POUND STRAWBERRIES, STEMS ON

1. Melt chocolate over low heat in pan or double boiler, or microwave.

2. Dip each strawberry into melted chocolate, holding it by the stem, and set on wax paper.

3. Chill in refrigerator until chocolate has hardened.

Yogurt Parfait

SERVES 1

Attractive, delicious, and sugar-free.

1 CONTAINER OF PLAIN YOGURT, DIVIDED
STRAWBERRIES, SLICED
BLUEBERRIES
GROUND CINNAMON

In a parfait glass (or comparable dish), place a layer of plain yogurt. Top with sliced strawberries. Add another layer of yogurt. Top with blueberries. Add one more layer of yogurt. Sprinkle with cinnamon.

Sugar-Free Cocoa

This recipe helps you get your chocolate fix without all the sugar. When you crave the taste of chocolate, pair it with the natural sweetness of milk.

8 OUNCES SKIM OR LOW-FAT MILK
1 TEASPOON UNSWEETENED COCOA POWDER
¼ TEASPOON GROUND CINNAMON

1. In a medium saucepan, heat milk to almost boiling.

2. Place cocoa powder in cup or mug. Add hot milk and mix well. Top with ground cinnamon.

Pear Crisp

With rich hints of nutmeg and cinnamon, this hot dish is best enjoyed on a cool night.

¼ CUP BUTTER OR MARGARINE, CUT IN CUBES
⅓ CUP UNCOOKED OATS
¼ CUP FLOUR
2 CUPS PEARS, CHOPPED
2 TEASPOONS FRESH LEMON JUICE
½ TEASPOON GRATED LEMON ZEST
¼ TEASPOON GROUND NUTMEG
½ TEASPOON GROUND CINNAMON

1. Preheat oven to 400°F.

2. In a medium bowl, combine butter, oats, and flour. Set aside.

3. In a large bowl, place pears, lemon juice, lemon zest, nutmeg, and cinnamon. Toss to coat.

4. Place the pears in a pie plate. Top with oat-butter-flour mixture.

5. Bake for 15 minutes or until done.

Fro-Yo Bars

Pulling one of these fruity bars out of the refrigerator will make you feel like a kid again.

1 CUP PLAIN, UNSWEETENED YOGURT
1 CUP BLUEBERRIES; OR STRAWBERRIES, HULLED AND SLICED;
    OR PEACHES, STONED AND SLICED

1. Place yogurt and fruit in blender and blend well.

2. Pour into molds and freeze overnight or at least 4 hours, until set.

Granita

YIELDS 6–12 SERVINGS

This chilly, refreshing dessert is a great way to cool your palate after a hot meal.

4 CUPS CUBED RIPE CANTALOUPE
1 CUP UNSWEETENED APPLE JUICE
¼ CUP LIME JUICE
1 CUP BLUEBERRIES, TO SERVE
1 CUP RASPBERRIES, TO SERVE

1. In blender, combine cantaloupe and juices; puree until smooth.

2. Pour into 9-by-13-inch pan and place in freezer.

3. About every half hour for 3 or 4 hours, take a fork and stir toward the center. Freeze at least 1 more hour.

4. Before serving, let stand at room temperature for about 20 minutes. Scoop into bowls and top with berries.

Incredibly Cool Quinoa Crêpes

One of the cooler inventions of modern times is quinoa flour. With it, you can make absolutely guilt-free crêpes and other treats.

COCONUT OIL FOR GREASING

¾ CUP QUINOA FLOUR

1½ TEASPOONS BAKING POWDER

¼ TEASPOON VANILLA EXTRACT

½ TEASPOON GROUND CINNAMON

⅔ CUP UNSWEETENED VANILLA ALMOND MILK

1 EGG

2 APPLES, CORED AND SLICED

½ TEASPOON CINNAMON

1. Preheat oven to 350° F.

2. Grease a large baking sheet with coconut oil. In a large bowl, thoroughly combine quinoa flour, baking powder, vanilla, cinnamon, milk, and egg. Drop batter by scant tablespoons onto baking sheet, leaving at least an inch between dollops.

3. Bake 15 to 20 minutes, until edges brown. Remove from the oven.

4. Meanwhile, place apples and cinnamon in a small stockpot and cover with water. Bring to a boil, cover, and simmer. Cook until apples are soft, about 10 minutes.

5. Top crêpes with apple mixture.

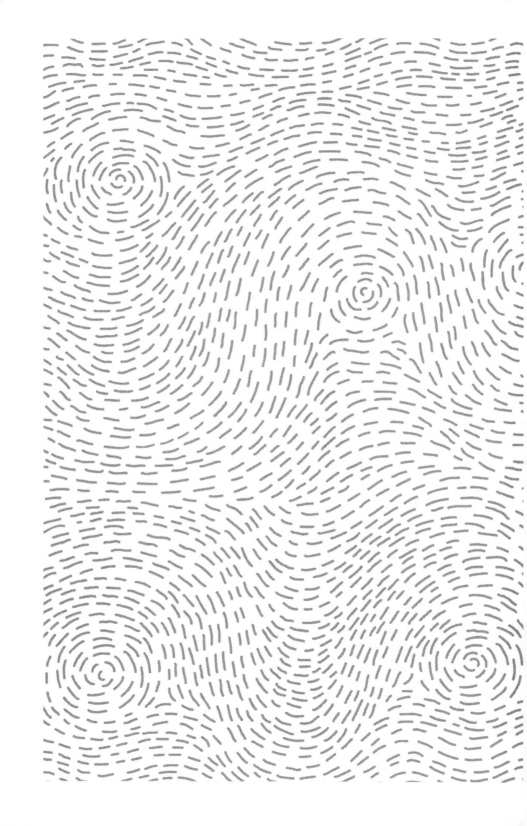

Resources

Cooking for the Specific Carbohydrate Diet, by Erica Kerwien (Berkeley, CA: Ulysses Press, 2013)

Eating Well on the Road, by Candy B. Harrington (Amazon Digital Services, 2013)

Jane Brody's Nutrition Book, by Jane Brody (New York: Bantam, 2013)

The Perricone Prescription, by Nicholas Perricone, MD (New York: Harper Collins, 2004)

The Self-Compassion Diet, by Jean Fain, LICSW, MSW (Boulder, CO: Sounds True, 2011)

Stop Aging, Start Living, by Alisa Bowman and Jeanette Graf, MD (New York: Three Rivers Press, 2007)

Sugar Shock! How Sweets and Simple Carbs Can Derail Your Life—and How You Can Get Back on Track, by Connie Bennett, CHHC, and Stephen Sinatra, MD (New York: Penguin, 2007)

Paula Simpson, nutritionist:
http://paulasimpson.com; www.twitter.com/@nutribeautiful
www.facebook.com/paulasimpson.nutritionist
www.youtube.com/user/glisodin1

Index